W9-BNC-379

Managed Care
What It Is and How It Works

Third Edition

Peter R. Kongstvedt, MD

JONES AND BARTLETT PUBLISHERS
Sudbury, Massachusetts
BOSTON   TORONTO   LONDON   SINGAPORE

World Headquarters

Jones and Bartlett Publishers
40 Tall Pine Drive
Sudbury, MA 01776
978-443-5000
info@jbpub.com
www.jbpub.com

Jones and Bartlett Publishers
Canada
6339 Ormindale Way
Mississauga, Ontario L5V 1J2
CANADA

Jones and Bartlett Publishers
International
Barb House, Barb Mews
London W6 7PA
UK

Jones and Bartlett's books and products are available through most bookstores and online booksellers. To contact Jones and Bartlett Publishers directly, call 800-832-0034, fax 978-443-8000, or visit our website, www.jbpub.com.

Substantial discounts on bulk quantities of Jones and Bartlett's publications are available to corporations, professional associations, and other qualified organizations. For details and specific discount information, contact the special sales department at Jones and Bartlett via the above contact information or send an email to specialsales@jbpub.com.

Production Credits

Publisher: Michael Brown
Production Director: Amy Rose
Associate Editor: Katey Birtcher
Editorial Assistant: Catie Heverling
Production Editor: Tracey Chapman
Production Assistant: Roya Millard
Marketing Manager: Sophie Fleck

Manufacturing and Inventory
 Control Supervisor: Amy Bacus
Composition: Arlene Apone
Cover Design: Brian Moore
Cover Image: ©Photos.com
Printing and Binding: Malloy, Inc.
Cover Printing: Malloy, Inc.

Library of Congress Cataloging-in-Publication Data
Kongstvedt, Peter R. (Peter Reid)
 Managed care : what it is and how it works / Peter R. Kongstvedt. -- 3rd ed.
  p. ; cm.
 Some of the chapters are adapted from previously published works by the same author.
 Includes bibliographical references and index.
 ISBN-13: 978-0-7637-5911-7 (pbk.)
 ISBN-10: 0-7637-5911-2 (pbk.)
 1. Managed care plans (Medical care)--United States. I. Title.
 [DNLM: 1. Managed Care Programs--organization & administration--United States. 2. Delivery of Health Care, Integrated--United States. W 130 AA1 K78m 2009]
 RA413.5.U5K655 2009
 362.1'0425--dc22

                    2008022680

6048

Printed in the United States of America
12 11 10 09   10 9 8 7 6 5 4 3 2

Dedication

To my wife Emily

New to This Edition

This edition contains very substantial revisions as well as updates to earlier material; for example, the introduction of new types of consumer-based health plans and services has practical implications throughout the book. Overall, this edition represents approximately 30–35 percent new or significantly revised material. Some revisions are subtle but meaningful (e.g., something that was once uncommon is now common and vice versa), whereas other changes are total (e.g., the section on Medicare was completely rewritten). Specific changes are outlined below.

Chapter 1–Added discussion of changes that took place in the past 5 years, including an extensive discussion of the "managed care backlash" that led to market shifts. Consumer-directed health plans (CDHPs) introduced.

Chapter 2–Updated to address CDHPs. Sections on types of managed care organizations (MCOs) and integrated delivery systems (IDSs) updated, including relative successes and declines of various types of MCOs and IDSs. Includes further discussion of CDHPs.

Chapter 3–Revisions discuss new approaches to provider networks, and additional discussion of hospital-based physicians. Revisions to reimbursement approaches, including new ones such as Medicare Severity Diagnosis-Related Groups (MS-DRGs). Section on pay-for-performance revised. Issues around consumerism and data transparency added.

Chapter 4–Approaches to care management, such as changes in approaches to disease management and basic utilization management, revised.

Chapter 5–Updates made around all core operational functions of MCOs, including significant updates to issues around claims management, member services, and sales and marketing. New issues around consumerism addressed.

Chapter 6–The new Medicare Modernization Act's prescription drug benefit and Medicare Advantage described. Section on Medicare fully rewritten. Section on Medicaid revised and updated.

Chapter 7–Section on state regulation of MCOs updated, including sections on state requirements and consumer protections. Section on the Health Insurance Portability and Accountability Act (HIPAA) extensively revised and rewritten, including requirements around electronic interactions, privacy, and information security. The section on the Employee Retirement Income Security Act (ERISA) also was revised to reflect new federal requirements. A brief discussion of the Consolidated Omnibus Reconciliation Act (COBRA) added. The section on accreditation of MCOs by the three major accreditation organizations was extensively revised, and the Healthcare Effectiveness Data and Information Set (HEDIS) updated. New material was added to discuss the Consumer Assessment of Healthcare Providers and Systems (CAHPS) survey.

Glossary–Revised by dropping some obsolete terms and adding new ones, and increasing the number of terms by nearly 25 percent.

Table of Contents

Preface

Since the second edition of *Managed Care: What It Is and How It Works* was published, managed care has continued its evolution. The "managed care backlash" described in Chapter 1 brought a reduction in some of the more active forms of managing care, as well as some movement in the marketplace from health maintenance organizations (HMOs) toward preferred provider organizations (PPOs) and newer forms of health plans. To be sure, HMOs remain an important element of the U.S. health care landscape, and PPOs and other types of health plans have adopted many of the more useful aspects that were once the domain of HMOs only, such as disease management. But in many ways, health care became a bit less "managed."

This, however, was accompanied by a rapid rise in healthcare costs, far exceeding that experienced in the years before the second edition of this book was published. There has been some moderation recently, but healthcare cost inflation remains two to three times higher than the general rate of inflation, and it's not likely to get much lower any time soon. Some of the factors behind cost inflation remain the same—hospitals are expensive places to run, for example. A few factors have declined; gross overutilization of inpatient stays is no longer the norm, for example, though increases in hospital charges has ensured that the cost for hospital care has not declined an equal amount. Some factors that used to be out of control, such as the cost of drugs, are now more in line with inflation in other parts of the system because of increasing use of generics, assisted by complex drug benefits plans. But new factors have emerged or grown, such as advances in technology and miniaturization, new biological drugs, and genetic testing, all of which contribute disproportionately to cost inflation. New diagnostic and therapeutic interventions continually appear, providing ever-expanding opportunities for medical interventions. And although physicians do not exhibit the same types of practice behaviors prevalent one and two decades ago, high levels of variability in practice across the country remain.

Because the medical care landscape is always changing, new approaches to managing cost, quality, and access will always be developed. Some of these will fail or lead to unintended consequences, whereas others will succeed and lead to still more changes. New approaches that start out in only one type of health plan migrate, if useful, to more mainstream types of health plans. This diffusion of effective approaches to managing healthcare cost and quality has always been a feature of the health sector in this country, and it continues today.

The path chosen by the United States, combining single-payer systems (i.e., Medicare, Medicaid, and other federal health programs) with a heavy reliance on private health insurance is unique in the industrialized world. The result includes rapid healthcare costs as a percentage of the gross domestic product, seen by most as a severe failing, but the result also includes advanced medical interventions and high access to care (i.e., little queuing and early treatment) that lead much of the rest of the world. The current system has also resulted in the greatest percentage of uninsured or underinsured citizens of any industrialized nation, and access to health care by the poor remains a problem. No simple solution exists to maintain the good while eliminating the bad.

The reality is that the healthcare delivery and financing system existing in the United States is incredibly complex, and that complexity is always accelerating, never slowing, or even increasing at a steady pace. As a result, it is possible to describe neither a steady state nor even a reliably predictable state. The notion of complexity is useful to bear in mind throughout the book. By doing so, the reader will maintain a sense of the true vibrancy of managed health care and will not fall into the trap of thinking that managed health care is monolithic or simplistic, or that there is only one way to do something.

Everything you read here is a reflection of health insurance and managed health care in 2008. An immediate and practical effect of the complex healthcare environment is that changes will continue to occur in this industry, and some of those changes will not have been anticipated in this book. Therefore, it is incumbent on the reader to ascertain for herself or himself the applicability and accuracy of the information presented, particularly in regard to federal and state laws. The fundamental concepts and attributes of managed health care nonetheless remain, regardless of such changes. The environmental forces that led to the creation and continued evolution of managed health care still exist and are, in many ways, even greater than in the past.

This edition contains very substantial revisions and updates to earlier material. The introduction of new types of consumer-based health plans and services has practical implications throughout the book. Approaches to provider networks have been revised to take into account not only new types of products but also new approaches to reimbursement and incentive systems. Care management continues to evolve, leading to revisions in that chapter. Operations in managed care have likewise evolved, leading to a revision of that chapter as well. External accreditation has become more sophisticated, also requiring considerable revisions. New laws and programs in Medicare required a complete rewriting of that section. Changes in federal laws and regulations meant that considerable updates and revisions were required, particularly around the Health Insurance Portability and Accountability Act (HIPAA). Finally, even the glossary was revised, dropping some obsolete terms and adding new ones, increasing the number of terms by nearly 25 percent.

Readers of *Managed Care: What It Is and How It Works, Third Edition,* should recognize the true vitality of managed care and not fall into the trap of thinking that it offers only one way to do something. Yet, in a field this complex, it is essential to begin with basic descriptions of the most prominent topics. This book does exactly that, as indicated by the following chapter summaries.

Chapter 1 focuses on the history and evolution of managed care. It provides the background necessary for readers to understand the nature of managed care as it exists today.

Chapter 2 describes the main types of managed care organizations (MCOs), integrated healthcare delivery systems, and new consumer-directed health plans. It also reviews the basic governance and management structure of health plans.

Chapter 3 is an overview of the healthcare delivery system. It describes the basic provider sectors—primary care physicians, specialty physicians, hospitals and other healthcare institutions, and ancillary services—and the way that managed care works within them. It also covers the topics of network development, network management, and reimbursement.

Chapter 4 explains how managed care actually manages health care. The basic components of care management include medical-surgical utilization management, case and disease management, management of pharmaceutical services, and quality management. Managed care is not simply about approving or denying payment for a healthcare service or contracting for favorable pricing; it is also about changing the way that health care is delivered.

Chapter 5 presents an account of the nonmedical operations of MCOs. The functions described include claims processing, information management, marketing and sales, member services, underwriting, and financial management. These are the foundational functions of any health plan, and they must operate properly for the plan to succeed.

Chapter 6 describes the Medicare and Medicaid programs and their increasing use of managed care to control costs, enhance the coordination of care, and improve its quality. The new Medicare Modernization Act created a new prescription drug benefit and redefined the various ways that managed care may be applied in Medicare through the Medicare Advantage program. The chapter also defines some of the differences between the two programs and indicates some of the ways that MCOs undertaking to serve Medicare and Medicaid populations must modify their operations to meet the programs' special requirements.

Chapter 7 focuses on the regulation of managed care. States continue to play a dominant role in the regulation of health plans, and a section on state requirements leads the chapter. Following that section is a discussion of several federal laws: HIPAA, which has hugely important implications for electronic interactions, privacy, and information security in all parts of the healthcare industry; the Employee Retirement Income Security Act (ERISA), which regulates self-funded health benefits plans; and, briefly, the Consolidated Omnibus Reconciliation Act (COBRA), which provides for continuation of coverage. Finally, the chapter describes the accreditation of MCOs by the three major accreditation organizations, and a brief discussion about two important sets of measurements: the Healthcare Effectiveness Data and Information Set (HEDIS) and the Consumer Assessment of Healthcare Providers and Systems (CAHPS) survey.

The book ends with a comprehensive glossary that provides definitions of terms commonly used in the managed care industry.

Much of the material found in this book has been distilled from the parent text of this series, *The Essentials of Managed Health Care, Fifth Edition.* Interested readers wanting additional information about most aspects of managed care are advised to consult that reference work, published by Jones & Bartlett in 2007. The main goal of this book is very simple—to provide its readers with a solid understanding of how health insurance and managed care actually works. If it succeeds in doing that, then some who are reading these words right now will be in a position to better contribute to the future evolution of this dynamic industry, thereby benefiting us all.

Peter Reid Kongstvedt
McLean, VA

Acknowledgments

Although I cannot name them all, since to do so would double the size of this book, I thank my many colleagues and friends in the managed care and consulting industries from whom I have learned so much over the years, and I look forward to continuing to do so. I also want to give sincere thanks to the many readers of previous editions of this book for their support, kind words, observations, and suggestions that have helped to strengthen the text.

About the Author

Dr. Peter Kongstvedt is a well-known and highly regarded independent national authority on health insurance and managed health care. He has 15 years of experience as a partner or senior executive in global consulting firms, and 13 years of operational experience in senior-most leadership positions at health plans, including managed care, health insurance, and Blue Cross Blue Shield organizations. He began his career practicing internal medicine.

Dr. Kongstvedt is the primary author and editor of several widely used books, including *The Essentials of Managed Health Care, Fifth Edition,* published by Jones & Bartlett in March 2007, and this book's predecessor, *Managed Care: What It Is and How It Works, Second Edition.* Dr. Kongstvedt is regarded as a thought leader in this industry sector, and he is a frequent contributor to various publications. He is also a frequent speaker and presenter at both industry conferences and client-sponsored events. Dr. Kongstvedt's client-focused activities include personal and strategic counsel to senior executives in various healthcare sectors, as well as working with boards of directors.

Dr. Kongstvedt received all of his education and training at the University of Wisconsin, and he is a board-certified internist. He may be reached through his web site at http://www.kongstvedt.com.

Keeping Current

Keeping current on trends and data presents significant challenges, particularly to trends and data presented in a book. However, there are several useful resources accessible via the Web that periodically provide updated data and trend information, and discussion on important health policy issues relevant to managed health care. The most useful of these follow.

(Note that all web addresses are current at the time of publication, but are always subject to change)

- The Centers for Medicare and Medicaid Services (CMS): http://www.cms.gov. (Free)
- The Office of the Actuary at CMS: http://www.cms.hhs.gov/NationalHealthExpendData/. (Free)
- The Centers for Disease Control and Prevention, National Center for Health Statistics: http://www.cdc.gov/nchs/. (Free)
- The Center for Studying Health System Change: http://www.hschange.com/. (Free)
- The Henry J. Kaiser Family Foundation (particularly their annual series on health insurance and healthcare marketplace trends): http://www.kff.org. (Free)
- The Agency for Healthcare Research and Quality: http://www.ahrq.gov. (Free)
- The annually updated Sanofi-Aventis Managed Care Digest Series: http://www.managedcaredigest.com. (Free with registration)
- HealthLeaders-InterStudy: http://home.healthleaders-interstudy.com. (Requires purchase)
- Health Affairs: http://www.healthaffairs.org/. (Requires subscription)

CHAPTER 1

The Origins of Managed Health Care

LEARNING OBJECTIVES

- Understand how managed care came into being
- Understand the forces that have shaped managed care in the past
- Understand the major obstacles to managed care historically
- Understand the major forces shaping managed care today

MANAGED CARE: THE EARLY YEARS (PRE–1970)

Sometimes cited as the first example of a health maintenance organization (HMO), the Western Clinic in Tacoma, Washington, began in 1910 to offer, exclusively through its own providers, a broad range of medical services in return for a premium payment of $0.50 per member per month. The program was available to lumber mill owners and their employees, and it served to ensure a flow of patients and revenues for the clinic. A similar program that was later developed in Tacoma expanded to 20 sites in Oregon and Washington.

In 1929, Dr. Michael Shadid established a rural farmers' cooperative health plan in Elk City, Oklahoma. Participating farmers purchased shares for $50 each to raise capital for a new hospital; in return, they received medical care at a discount. Because of the medical community's opposition to this new concept, Shadid lost his membership in the county medical society and was threatened with suspension of his license to practice medicine. Some 20 years later, however, he was vindicated through an out-of-court settlement in his favor of an antitrust suit against the county and state medical societies. In 1934, the Farmers Union assumed control of both the hospital and the health plan.

As Starr noted,[1] health insurance itself is of relatively recent origin. In 1929, Baylor Hospital in Texas agreed to provide some 1,500 teachers with prepaid care at its hospital, an arrangement that represented the origins of Blue Cross. The program was subsequently expanded to include other employers and hospitals, initially through single hospital plans. Starting in 1939, a number of state medical societies, such as that in California, created Blue Shield plans to cover physician services. At the time, commercial health insurance was not a factor.

The formation of the various Blue Cross and Blue Shield plans, as well as the beginning of many HMOs, in the midst of the Great Depression came about not because consumers were demanding insurance against the risk of medical expenses or because nonphysician entrepreneurs were seeking to establish a business, but rather because providers wanted to maintain and enhance patient revenues. Many of these developments were threatening to organized medicine. In 1932, the American Medical Association (AMA) adopted a strong position against prepaid group practices, favoring instead indemnity-type insurance that protects the policyholder from expenses by reimbursement. The AMA took this stance in response to the prepaid group practices in existence at the time (although few in number) and to the findings in 1932 of the Committee on the Cost of Medical Care—a highly visible private group of leaders from medicine, dentistry, public health, consumers, and so forth—that recommended the expansion of group practice as an efficient health care delivery system. The AMA's opposition set the tone for continued state and local medical society resistance to prepaid group practice at the state and local medical society levels.

The period immediately surrounding World War II saw the formation of several HMOs, some of which remain prominent today. They represent a diversity of origins, as the initial impetus came variously from employers seeking benefits for their employees, providers seeking patient revenues, consumers seeking access to improved and affordable health care, and even a housing lending agency seeking a reduction in the number of foreclosures. The following are examples of early HMOs:

- The Kaiser Foundation Health Plans were started in 1937 by Dr. Sidney Garfield at the request of the Kaiser construction company. The purpose was to finance medical care for workers who were building an aqueduct in the southern California desert to transport water from the Colorado River to Los Angeles and, subsequently, for workers who were constructing the Grand Coulee Dam in Washington State. A similar program was established in 1942 at Kaiser shipbuilding plants in the San Francisco Bay area.

- In 1937, the Home Owner's Loan Corporation organized the Group Health Association (GHA) in Washington, D.C., to reduce the number of mortgage defaults by families who had large medical expenses. It was a non-profit consumer cooperative, with the board of directors elected periodically by the enrollees. The District of Columbia Medical Society opposed the formation of GHA, seeking to restrict hospital admitting privileges for GHA physicians and threatening to expel those physicians from the medical society. A bitter antitrust battle ensued that culminated in the U.S. Supreme Court's ruling in favor of GHA. In 1994, GHA was facing insolvency despite an enrollment of some 128,000 members. Humana Health Plans, a for-profit publicly traded corporation, acquired GHA but has since disbanded it. The membership now belongs to the Kaiser Foundation Health Plan of the Mid-Atlantic.

- In 1944, in response to the needs of New York City seeking coverage for its employees, the Health Insurance Plan (HIP) of Greater New York was formed.

- In 1947, consumers in Seattle organized 400 families, who contributed $100 each, to form the Group Health Cooperative of Puget Sound. Predictably, the Kings County Medical Society opposed the cooperative.

These pioneer prepaid group practices encountered varying degrees of opposition from local medical societies.

The early independent practice association (IPA) model HMOs, which contract with physicians in independent fee-for-service practice, were developed as a way of competing with group-practice-based HMOs. The basic structure was created in 1954, when the San Joaquin County Medical Society in California formed the San Joaquin Medical Foundation in response to competition from the Kaiser Foundation Health Plans. The San Joaquin Medical Foundation established a relative value fee schedule for paying physicians, heard grievances against physicians, and monitored the quality of health care. It received a license from the state to accept a set monthly fee (i.e., capitation payment) to provide for each person enrolled in the plan all the health care services that he or she needed, making it the first IPA model HMO. Only in later years did nonprovider entrepreneurs form for-profit HMOs in significant numbers.

THE ADOLESCENT YEARS OF MANAGED CARE: 1970–1985

Through the 1960s and into the early 1970s, HMOs played only a modest role in the financing and delivery of health care. Although they were a significant presence in a few communities, such as the Seattle area and parts of California, the total number of HMOs nationwide in 1970 fell somewhere in the 30s, the exact number depending on the definition. From then until the early to mid-1990s, HMOs expanded at an ever-increasing rate. However, beginning in the early to mid-1990s, HMOs consolidated through mergers and acquisitions, resulting in a decline in the number of such plans beginning in the late 1990s, as discussed later in this chapter.

The major boost to the HMO movement during this period was the enactment in 1973 of the federal Health Maintenance Organization Act. That act authorized start-up funding and, more important, ensured access to the employer-based health insurance market. The act evolved from discussions that Dr. Paul Ellwood had in 1970 with the officials of the U.S. Department of Health, Education and Welfare (which later became the U.S. Department of Health and Human Services). Ellwood had participated in designing the Health Planning Act of 1966 during the presidency of Lyndon Johnson.

Ellwood, sometimes referred to as the father of the modern HMO movement, was asked in the early years of the Nixon administration to devise ways of constraining the increases in the Medicare budget. His conversations with federal officials led to a proposal to reimburse HMOs for Medicare beneficiaries' health care through a capitation system (a proposal that was not enacted until 1982) and laid the groundwork for what became the HMO Act of 1973. The emphasis on HMOs at this time reflected the perspective that the fee-for-service system, by rewarding physicians for providing more services rather than for providing appropriate services, incorporated the wrong incentives. Also, the term "health maintenance organization" was coined then as a substitute for prepaid group practice, principally because it had greater public appeal.

The main features of the HMO Act were these:

- It made grants and loans available for the planning and start-up phases of new HMOs as well as for service area expansions for existing HMOs.
- It overrode state laws that restricted the development of HMOs if the HMOs met federal requirements for certification.
- Most important of all, it required employers with 25 or more employees that offered indemnity coverage also to offer up to two different types of federally qualified HMO options if the plans made a formal request. For workers under collective bargaining agreements, the union had to agree to the offering. Many HMOs were reluctant to exercise the mandate, fearing that making such a request would antagonize employers and cause them to discourage employees from enrolling. However, many other HMOs used the dual-choice provision to at least advertise themselves to employer groups.

The statute also established the process under which HMOs could elect to obtain federal qualification. Unlike state licensure, which is mandatory, federal qualification had always been at the discretion of the individual HMO. To obtain federal qualification, HMOs had to satisfy a series of requirements, such as meeting minimum benefit package standards set forth in the act, demonstrating that their provider networks were adequate, having a quality assurance system in place, complying with standards of financial stability, and establishing an enrollee grievance system. Some states emulated these requirements and adopted them for all HMOs that were licensed in the state, regardless of federal qualification status.

Plans that requested federal qualification did so for four principal reasons. First, qualification represented a "seal of approval" that was helpful in marketing. Second, the required offering of HMO options ensured that HMOs that were federally qualified would have access to the employer market. Third, the override of state laws—important in some states but not in others—applied only to federally qualified HMOs. Fourth, only those HMOs that obtained federal qualification could receive the federal grants and loans that were available during the early years of the act.

The slowness of the federal government in issuing the regulations implementing the act also delayed HMO development. Employers knew that they would have to contract with federally qualified plans. Even those that supported the mandate had to wait until the government determined which plans would be qualified and established the processes for implementing the dual-choice provisions. In 1977, however, at the beginning of the Carter administration, issuance of the regulations became a priority, and rapid growth ensued.

Federal qualification is no longer law, but its impact on the early establishment and growth of HMOs cannot be underestimated. Politically, several other aspects of this history are noteworthy. For example, although differences arose on specifics, congressional support for legislation promoting HMO development came from both political parties. Also, there was no widespread state opposition to the federal override of restrictive state laws. In addition, most employers did not actively oppose the dual-choice requirements, although many disliked being required to contract with HMOs by the federal government. Perhaps most interesting of all was the generally positive interaction between the public sector and the private sector, with government fostering HMO development both through its regulatory processes and its purchase of health care coverage under its employee benefits programs.

Among the other managed care developments that took place during the 1970s and early 1980s was the creation of the preferred provider organization (PPO), a plan that contracts with a limited number of independent providers to obtain services for its members at a discount. It is generally believed that the PPO originated in Denver, where, in the early 1970s, Samuel Jenkins, a vice president at the benefits consulting firm, the Martin E. Segal Company, negotiated discounts with hospitals on behalf of the company's Taft-Hartley trust fund clients. Utilization review also evolved outside the HMO setting between 1970 and 1985, although it has earlier origins:

- In 1959, Blue Cross of Western Pennsylvania, the Allegheny County Medical Society Foundation, and the Hospital Council of Western Pennsylvania performed retrospective analyses of hospital claims to identify utilization that was significantly above average.
- Around 1970, California's Medicaid program began to require preadmission authorization for routine hospitalizations and concurrent review in conjunction with medical care foundations in the state, starting with the Sacramento Foundation for Medical Care. Such foundations were not-for-profit organizations usually created by local organized medicine or medical societies for purposes of conducting utilization review and, later, creating independent practice association types of HMOs.
- The 1972, Social Security Amendments authorized the federal Professional Standards Review Organization (PSRO) program to review the appropriateness of care provided to Medicare and Medicaid beneficiaries. Although its effectiveness has been debated, the PSRO program established an organizational infrastructure and data capacity on which both the public and

private sectors could rely. In time, the PSRO was replaced by the Peer Review Organization (PRO), itself in turn replaced by the quality improvement organization (QIO), which continues to provide oversight of clinical services on behalf of the federal and many state governments. Although the methods used by these organizations evolved along with their acronyms, their focus remained essentially the same.

- In the 1970s, a handful of large corporations initiated programs for preauthorization and concurrent review for inpatient care.

Developments in indemnity insurance, mostly during the 1980s, included (1) encouraging persons with conventional insurance to obtain second opinions before undergoing elective surgery and (2) adopting "large case management" (i.e., the coordination of services for persons with conditions that require expensive medical care, such as selected accident patients, cancer patients, and very low birth weight infants). Also during the 1980s, work site wellness programs became more prevalent as employers, to varying degrees and in varying ways, instituted such programs as the following:

- Screening (e.g., for hypertension and diabetes)
- Health risk appraisal
- Exercise promotion (whether by providing access to gyms, conveniently located showers, or running paths, or by simply providing information)
- Stress reduction
- Classes (e.g., smoking cessation, weight lifting)
- Nutrition, including the serving of healthy food in the cafeteria
- Weight loss
- Mental health counseling

MANAGED CARE GROWS UP: 1985 TO 2000

The period between 1985 and 2000 saw a combination of innovation, maturation, and restructuring. Growth in HMOs was rapid and reached a peak in 2000 but began to decline after that, as will be discussed in a later section.

Innovation

In many communities, physicians and hospitals collaborated to form integrated delivery systems (IDSs). These had two principal forms. The first form was a single legal entity made up of hospitals and hospital-employed physicians. The other form was a physician–hospital organization (PHO), principally as a vehicle for contracting with managed care organizations. Typically, most PHOs sought to enter into fee-for-service arrangements with HMOs and PPOs, although for a period, a number sought full-risk capitation. Full-risk capitation, as discussed in Chapter 3, involves the IDS or PHO accepting a fixed amount of money per member per month for all health care expenses. However, with the failure of many such full-risk arrangements in the years 1999 and 2000, acceptance of full-risk capitation has sharply declined. Further, productivity problems that arose when physicians went from private practice to being employed caused a number of hospital-based IDSs to abandon the physician employment model.

For several reasons, PHOs did not become important elements of the managed care environment. Their reimbursement systems, for example, did not support the primary managed care goals of cost containment and efficient care. The typical PHO allowed all physicians with admitting privileges at the hospital to participate in the plan rather than selecting the more efficient ones, and it also required physicians to use the hospital for outpatient services (e.g., laboratory tests) that might have been available at lower cost elsewhere, hurting its price competitiveness. Finally, some PHOs were poorly organized, had inadequate information systems, operated under inexperienced management, or lacked the necessary capital for investment. In the end, PHOs with these kinds of problems were not able to sustain the financial risks.

The development of carve-out companies—organizations that have specialized provider networks that offer specific services, such as mental health care, management of a particular disease (e.g., congestive heart failure, diabetes), chiropractic treatment, and dental services—occurred during this period. The carve-out companies market their services primarily to HMOs and large self-insured employers. In recent years, some of the large health plans that contracted for such specialty services have reintegrated them back into the main company (so called carve-in or in-sourcing). One reason for the reintegration was the view that carved-out services made it difficult to coordinate services (e.g., between physical and mental health).

Advances in computer technology have made other innovations possible. Vastly improved computer programs, marketed by private firms or developed by managed care plans for internal use, can generate statistical profiles of the services rendered by physicians. These profiles serve not only as a means to assess the efficiency and the quality of the care that each physician provides but also as a basis for the adjustment of payment levels to providers who are paid under capitation or risk-sharing arrangements that reflect the severity of illness among each provider's patient group.

Computer technology is responsible for a virtual revolution in the processing of medical and drug claims. The increasingly widespread use of electronic processing rather than paper submission and manual entry has substantially lowered administrative costs and broadened access to far superior information; when dispensing a prescription, for example, the pharmacist can now receive information about eligibility of the member for coverage, amount of copay or coinsurance required on a drug-by-drug basis, and potential adverse effects and interactions. Management information systems can be expected to improve in the next few years as providers, almost universally, submit claims electronically. Requirements under the Health Insurance Portability and Accountability Act of 1996 (HIPAA) for administrative simplification have accelerated the movement toward inexpensive electronic interchange for the basic transactions in managed care, including:

- Claims
- Claims status
- Authorizations
- Eligibility checking
- Payment

Maturation

Maturation during this period can be seen from several vantage points. The first was the extent of HMO and PPO growth. In the mid-1980s, HMOs grew fastest, but by the early 1990s, PPOs began to grow even faster. By the late 1990s, HMOs actually began to decline, whereas PPOs continued to grow. During the entire period, conventional health insurance continually declined. In parallel to enrollment trends in the commercial sector, Medicare HMO enrollment grew from 1.3 to 6.3 million between 1990 and 1999.

Another phenomenon was the maturation of external quality oversight activities. Starting in 1991, the National Committee for Quality Assurance (NCQA; see Chapter 7) began to accredit HMOs. The NCQA was launched by the HMOs' trade association in 1979 but became independent in 1991, with the majority of board seats being held by employer, union, and consumer representatives. Many employers are requiring or strongly encouraging NCQA accreditation of the HMOs with which they contract, and accreditation came to replace federal qualification as the seal of approval. NCQA, which initially focused only on

HMOs, has evolved with the market, for example, to encompass mental health carve-outs, PPOs, physician credentialing verification organizations, and others. In addition to NCQA, other bodies that accredit managed care plans have also developed, as described in Chapter 7.

Performance measurement systems (report cards) continue to evolve, the most prominent being the Health Care Effectiveness Data and Information Set (HEDIS), which was developed by the NCQA. The HEDIS data set has evolved and grown on a regular basis, and a list of current HEDIS measures is found in Chapter 7. Other forms of report cards have appeared since then and continue to develop as the market demands increasing levels of sophistication.

Another form of maturation is the focus of cost management efforts, which used to be almost exclusively inpatient hospital utilization. Practice patterns changed during this period, and inpatient utilization declined. Although inpatient utilization still receives considerable scrutiny, greater attention began to be paid to ambulatory services such as prescription drugs, diagnostics, and care by specialists. Perhaps even more important is that the high concentration of costs in a small number of patients with chronic conditions resulted in significantly more attention being paid to disease management, as discussed in Chapter 4.

Restructuring

Perhaps the most dramatic development was the restructuring that began in the late 1980s, reflecting the interplay between managed care, the health care delivery system, and the overall health care marketplace. The definition distinctions blurred as payers created hybrid products, as will be discussed in Chapter 2. Staff- and group-model HMOs declined in number and formed IPA components, and in some cases even eliminated the medical group or staff model itself. HMOs expanded their offerings to include PPO and point-of-service (POS) products, and some PPOs obtained HMO licenses. HMOs also found themselves contracting with employers on a self-funded rather than an at-risk basis, meaning that the risk for medical costs remained with the employer. The major commercial health insurance companies also dramatically increased their involvement in managed care by both acquiring local health plans and starting up HMOs and PPOs. In short, the managed care environment became even more complicated.

Another change was in the role of the primary care physician (PCP), who assumed responsibility for overseeing the care of the HMO member. In a traditional HMO, the role of the PCP has been to manage a patient's medical care, including access to specialty care. This proved to be a mixed blessing for PCPs, who sometimes felt caught between pressures to reduce costs on the one hand, and the need to satisfy the desires of consumers on the other. The growing popularity of PPOs as compared with HMOs appears to have led to a shift away from PCP-based plans during this time. In some HMOs, for example, the requirement for PCP authorization to access specialty services, known as the "gatekeeper" requirement, began to be eliminated. That said, many plans (including PPOs) still provide for lower copays if a member receives care from a PCP rather than a specialist.

Finally, consolidation was, and continues to be, notable among both health care plans and providers. Among physicians, there continues a slow but clear movement away from solo practice and toward group practice. As for hospitals, a substantial amount of consolidation on a regional or local level occurred, creating large local and regional systems. Consolidation in the provider sector occurred largely in the mid- to late 1990s and continues today, although at a slower rate.

Health plan consolidation has been constant during this period and continues today. Smaller local health plans have been acquired or, in some cases, have ceased operations because of a number of forces. Large employers with employees who are spread geographically have generally been moving toward national companies at the expense of local health plans. For smaller plans, the financial strain of having to continually upgrade computer systems and other technology can become excessive. Smaller plans may also find themselves unable to negotiate the same discounts as larger competitors; smaller plans in unique markets, such as in rural areas or where physician loyalty is high, may continue to thrive, but beginning in this period and continuing today, it is getter harder for smaller plans to succeed.

Even larger health plans have been targets for acquisition, primarily in the for-profit sector. During this period, some, but not all, Blue Cross Blue Shield plans converted to for-profit status. Blue Cross Blue Shield plans, which had been dominant, began to lose market share during this time. However, they adapted to the changing market, and by the mid-1990s had begun to regain it in their managed care products.

MANAGED CARE IN RECENT TIMES: 2000–2007

The economic boom of the mid- to late 1990s changed the dynamics in the managed health care industry. As a result of unemployment dropping below 4%, corporate profits being strong, and the economy growing, employers found it increasingly necessary to compete for employees. The anti–managed care rhetoric of political campaigns, combined with media "horror stories," helped fuel negative public sentiment about managed care as discussed in the next section. The result was a movement away from traditional managed care and toward less managed types of health plans.

HMOs declined to 66.1 million in 2004 but rose again to 77.7 million by 2006, fueled in large part by increasing Medicare enrollment. Medicare HMOs themselves had declined to 4.6 million by 2003 because HMOs exited the market after sustaining significant losses, but they too rose again to 8.8 million by 2007 (not counting an additional 17 million Medicare beneficiaries enrolled in stand-alone prescription drug plans). By comparison, approximately 81 million people enrolled in PPOs by 2006. However, insurance carriers sell hybrid products that combine elements of HMOs and PPOs, making statistical compilations difficult.

Market growth in the Blue Cross Blue Shield system has been considerable as a result of many factors, including its generally broad provider networks, the managed care backlash (discussed in the next section), and the Blue's improved ability to offer national accounts as compared with the prior decade. In any given state, the Blue plan often has the highest market penetration of any health plan

Consolidation of payer companies continued to the point that by 2007, four commercial for-profit companies accounted for over 45% of covered individuals: CIGNA, Aetna, United Health Care, and WellPoint. WellPoint itself is made up largely of for-profit Blue Cross Blue Shield plans, though it also has non-Blue commercial business. Consolidation also continued in the not-for-profit sector, again primarily (but not exclusively) in Blue Cross and Blue Shield plans.

The Managed Care Backlash

Anti–managed care sentiment, commonly referred to as the "managed care back-lash," became a defining force in the industry in the 1990s. Political speeches, movies and television shows, news articles, and even cartoons increasingly began to portray managed care in an unflattering light. There were several reasons for this.

Because managed care had significantly lower costs than traditional health plans, it became a dominant form of health care coverage when many employers put their employees (and dependents) into managed care as their only type of coverage. As more and more people were enrolled in managed care plans, the number of problems rose as well. Many individuals did not want to be in a managed care plan but had no choice (or no affordable choice).

Some of the problems were more like irritants, such as mistakes in paperwork or claims processing in health plans with information technology (IT) systems that were unable to handle the load. Other problems were highly emotional, though not actually a threat to health, such as denial of coverage for care that was genuinely not medically necessary (e.g., an unnecessary diagnostic test). Finally, a major source of contention with many consumers was the requirement that they obtain prior authorization from their PCP to access specialty care. A few problems, however, were real, or at least potential threats to health, such as denial of coverage for truly necessary medical care or difficulties in accessing care. Although uncommon, problems of this nature quickly generate bad publicity, and bad news travels fast.

The managed care industry was not simply an innocent victim of bad publicity, though. As managed care companies grew, their ability actually to manage the delivery system was often poor. Where decisions on clinical issues were once done with active involvement of medical directors, the rapidly growing health plans became increasingly bureaucratic. Rapid growth also led to greater inconsistencies in decision making about benefits coverage. The public's perception that decisions were being made by "bean counters" or faceless clerks may not have been completely fair or accurate, but neither was it completely inaccurate. Decision-making authority was often delegated and not necessarily done with a sense of compassion or flexibility.

Perhaps the most serious charge leveled against the managed care industry was the accusation that health plans *deliberately* refused to pay for necessary care to generate profits and make executives and shareholders rich, something that was emphasized by media stories of multi-million-dollar compensation packages for senior executives in the managed health care industry. Of course, financial incentives drive almost all aspects of health care to varying degrees, but this was a particularly damaging charge that health plans faced.

One result of the backlash were new consumer protections at the state or federal level, or at least the threat of such legislation. For example, many states passed legislation—the so-called prudent lay person rule—guaranteeing payment for emergency services if the symptoms could reasonably have been interpreted as an emergency—for example, chest pain, even if it turned out to be indigestion. States also passed bills instituting state-supervised independent appeals processes in the event of a medical denial. Finally, several unsuccessful attempts were made at the federal level to pass a so-called patient bill of rights.

Another frequently cited reason for the managed care backlash is American's desire for choice. People simply do not want to be told that they cannot go to any provider and still receive full coverage for their care. This attitude caused many HMOs to expand their networks aggressively and also drove the shift from traditional HMOs to less restrictive forms of coverage such as PPOs. The traditional indemnity type of health insurance remained unaffordable, however. Another example of the movement toward less restrictive forms of coverage is that a number of HMOs abandoned the PCP model (the so-called gatekeeper model discussed in Chapter 2) to one of "open access," allowing members to access any provider in the network, though usually with lower copays for primary care than for specialty care.

During this time, the managed care industry kept pointing out the good things that it was doing for members, such as coverage for preventive services and drugs, the absence of lifetime coverage limits, coverage of highly expensive care, and so forth. But it was of no use; as a reporter for a major newspaper once said to one of this chapter's authors, "We don't report safe airplane landings at LaGuardia either."

The managed care backlash has now become mostly an echo. The volume of HMO jokes has declined, news stories about coverage restrictions or withheld care are now uncommon, and there is little or no state or federal attention paid to placing restrictions on managed care plans.

The Return of Health Cost Inflation

The rapid increases in health care costs experienced in the late 1980s and early 1990s had slowed considerably by the mid-1990s, but health cost inflation returned by the turn of the century. Managed care had been a significant contributor to holding down the rate of rise, but many of the fundamental reasons for increased health care costs remain today. The health economy is too complex to say that increasing health care costs are due to any single reason, or even a small number of reasons. Where health cost inflation was once caused as much by unnecessary utilization as by anything else, other factors have always been present. The loosening of some of the controls traditionally associated with managed care, combined with richer benefits, certainly contributed to rising health costs, but numerous other factors have also been in play. Examples of other such factors are the following:

- Drug therapy advances and prescription drug costs
- Increasing numbers of outpatient procedures
- Continuing large variations in medical practice behavior
- High incomes for some types of providers (regardless of efficiency or quality)
- Greater consumer demands on the health care system
- Our high rate of lawsuits, causing physicians to practice defensive medicine
- High administrative costs
- Shifting demographics, including the aging of the population
- Expectations for a long and healthy life, regardless of costs
- The cost of complying with government mandates

These usual suspects are not the only ones pushing health cost inflation, however. Two relatively new categories are establishing themselves as major drivers of cost inflation: (1) rapidly developing (and usually expensive) medical technology, and (2) genomics. Examples of new medical technology are the implantable cardiac defibrillator, drug-eluting vascular stents, new orthopedic implants, and miniaturization of devices, to name a few. In the arena of genomics, the appearance of so-called specialty pharmacy, injectable drugs that are proteins manufactured through DNA replication, has led to treatments that may not be used frequently but that are hugely expensive when they are, commonly costing in excess of $10,000 per patient per year. The discovery of various alleles (i.e., genes) for cancer that help guide physicians as to the best therapy depending on the genetic profile (e.g., for breast cancer) are all adding to cost inflation.

MANAGED HEALTH CARE TODAY

At the same time that health benefits costs began rising, the economy began to soften, and increasingly, US companies have become confronted with competition from abroad—from companies that do not face the insurance costs of their American counterparts. These two forces led not to a return to traditional managed care, but rather to an increase in cost sharing with consumers through higher payroll deductions for health insurance premiums and, more important, in the form of changes in the benefits. Levels of copayments and coinsurance have been rising and in many cases have become more complex. For example, physician office visit copays that were once commonly $5 are now $20 or more, or may now be coinsurance (in which the consumer pays a percentage of the cost rather than a fixed copayment), as well as a deductible (in which the consumer must pay all costs until the deductible has been met). Pharmacy benefits that were once simple copays now have widely differing levels of copayment tiering and significant deductibles. Ironically, cost sharing was the primary method of cost control available to indemnity insurance prior to the advent of managed health care.

The most recent significant development is the rise of the consumer-directed health plan (CDHP), including such variants as health savings accounts (HSAs) and other types of high-deductible health plans (HDHPs) as more fully described in Chapter 2. Two hallmarks of CDHPs are greater cost sharing by consumers, combined with the notion that consumer choice and consumer accountability have greatly increased in importance. CDHPs are also associated with pretax funds to help pay for some costs. Health plans are working to better provide information to consumers about the quality and cost of the care they are seeking, and to help consumers choose physicians and hospitals and better understand their health care options. Informing consumers through information or "data transparency" and providing financial budgeting tools and other forms of information are currently the focus of much effort in all health plans, not just CDHPs.

The other major development was passage of the Medicare Modernization Act (MMA). In addition to a new drug benefit for Medicare beneficiaries, the MMA created new forms of Medicare managed care, collectively referred to as Medicare Advantage. Likewise, many states continue to turn to managed care for their Medicaid programs for low-income individuals. Both Medicare and Medicaid are discussed further in Chapter 6.

Managed care has not simply gone to higher cost sharing combined with improved information to assist in decision making. For example, new pay-for-performance programs are being tested and implemented to align financial incentives for providers with quality goals, as discussed in Chapter 3. Practice behavior by physicians continues to change, and as care management becomes more sophisticated, managed care companies have placed more emphasis on chronic and/or highly expensive medical conditions, with less focus on routine care, as discussed in Chapter 4.

CONCLUSION

The health care sector in the United States is highly dynamic. The roots of managed health care, and health insurance in general, are many. The continued growth and evolution of managed health care is affected by the health sector economy, marketplace needs, legal and regulatory requirements, changes in health care delivery, consumer demands, politics, and many other forces, all of which interact with each other. What started out with simple roots has become complex, and will only become more so.

NOTES

1. P. Starr, *The Social Transformation of American Medicine* (New York: Basic Books, 1982).

This chapter is adapted from P.D. Fox and P. R. Kongstvedt, "Chapter 1: An Overview of Managed Care," in *The Essentials of Managed Health Care*, 5th edition, ed. P. R. Kongstvedt (Sudbury, MA: Jones & Bartlett Publishers, 2007).

CHAPTER 2

Types of Managed Care Organizations and Integrated Health Care Delivery Systems

LEARNING OBJECTIVES

- Understand the basic managed care organization models
- Understand the differences between models
- Understand the principal services offered by managed care organizations
- Understand the primary structural components of managed care organizations

INTRODUCTION

Defining the different types of managed care organizations (MCOs) is an ever-evolving challenge. Fifteen or more years ago, it was relatively easy to distinguish among different types of MCOs. Health maintenance organizations (HMOs), preferred provider organizations (PPOs), and point-of-service (POS) health plans were distinct types of organizations and were identified as such. And 15 years ago, there was no such thing as a consumer-directed health plan (CDHP). The term "managed care" itself, once used to describe nearly all the activities covered in this book, is now used less frequently because of the negative association, as discussed in Chapter 1. In fact, many companies have even gone back to using the older term "health insurance," even if they still operate like managed care plans in many ways, whereas other organizations refer to themselves by the rather vague term "health plan."

Clear distinctions between types of health plans have become progressively blurred, and organizational elements that had appeared previously in only one type of MCO have found their way into other types of MCOs. As a result, it is now unusual to find health plans that are pure examples of a type, and those that do exist are frequently organizations that serve only small, well-defined market areas (i.e., niche organizations)—though there are some notable exceptions, such as Kaiser Permanente. More often, a seemingly pure MCO will be a subsidiary of a larger health plan or insurance company that offers other types of MCOs to the same market.

It is instructive to examine the different forms of MCOs, even if the boundaries between those forms are no longer clear in today's market. Although most MCOs have elements of more than one MCO type, they often still fall into one of the standard classifications. Finally, it is instructive to examine different types of integrated health care delivery systems (IDSs),* which are organized groups of providers. Various types of IDSs were initially formed in response to managed care, and they still carry out that purpose but may have other uses as well. The first portion of this chapter will focus on different types of MCOs, and the second part will focus on IDSs. And as always, there may be overlap.

In all cases, the first issue to address is what mechanism is used to bear risk for medical costs. At its core, the fundamental concept of pooling people's dollars into a single "risk pool" is used to spread the risk around. Everyone in a particular risk pool—employees of a company, for example—pay the same amount in, but the medical costs for each individual or family are not the same.

BEARING RISK FOR MEDICAL COSTS

Contrary to popular belief, an insurance company or MCO does not necessarily bear all the financial risks associated with the medical costs of its clients or members, and how it is structured or operates may be independent of the issue of fi-

---

* There is no reason that the *H* doesn't get used in this abbreviation other than the fact that "IDS" rolls off the tongue better. IDS is the term commonly used.

nancial risk for medical costs. There are three broad types of risk bearing from the standpoint of who pays the cost for health insurance (see Figure 2–1 and Exhibit 2–1): (1) government programs, (2) insurance, and (3) self-funded programs. Government programs and self-funded programs are briefly described here and discussed further in Chapters 6 and 7. Insurance is also briefly described here and is discussed throughout the entire book.

Government Programs

In the United States, the federal and state governments actually provide or finance more than 40 percent of health care. Government programs include Medicare for the elderly and disabled, Medicaid for the poor, military programs (both direct care by military providers and the TRICARE program under the Civilian Health and Medical Program of the Uniformed Services [CHAMPUS]), the Veterans Administration, the U.S. Public Health Service, and the Indian Health Service, among others. Some programs may incorporate only a few managed care features, others incorporate several features, and still others incorporate all features.

The most important government programs are those that entitle certain eligible individuals to receive benefits from the government. These are called entitlement programs, and the primary examples are Medicare and Medicaid. The Centers for Medicare & Medicaid Services (CMS), a branch of the U.S. Department of Health and Human Services, administers Medicare, which provides health insurance for the elderly and for many individuals with end-stage renal disease. The states manage the Medicaid programs, which receive state and federal

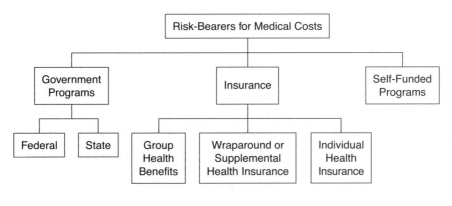

FIGURE 2–1 Risk Bearers for Medical Costs

EXHIBIT 2–1

Risk Bearers for Medical Costs

1. Government Programs
   - Government (federal and/or state) bears risk for medical expenses unless it has contracted risk out to private health plans. Ultimately government agencies and taxpayers bear the risk.
   - Examples: Medicaid, Medicare, Federal Employees Health Benefit Program.
2. Insurance
   - Insurance company bears risk for medical expenses.
   - State governments set regulations regarding premiums charged to consumers or employers, benefits covered under policy, and privacy of health information.
   - Examples: Group health benefits plans, wraparound or supplemental health insurance, and individual health insurance.
3. Self-Funded Health Benefits Plans
   - Employers bear risk for medical expenses but usually purchase reinsurance to provide coverage for catastrophically expensive cases.
   - No state regulation. Employer must comply with federal requirements under ERISA.*

*ERISA = Employee Retirement Income Security Act; see Chapter 7.

funds and provide health insurance to the poor and many disabled or institutionalized individuals.

Managed care techniques have been applied to all types of government programs, and there are, in fact, specific types of MCOs developed for Medicare and Medicaid. There is also a type of IDS called a provider-sponsored organization (PSO) that is able to contract directly with CMS to provide prepaid medical services to an enrolled group of Medicare beneficiaries. However, although a few PSOs still exist, most failed, and they are now quite rare.

In all government entitlement programs, the risk for medical expenses is borne by state and/or federal government agencies and, ultimately, the taxpayers. This may be confusing to some individuals in the case of Medicare because CMS contracts with private health plans, referred to as intermediaries, to administer the benefits of the traditional Medicare program. In other words, the intermediary processes the claims of Medicare beneficiaries but does so only as an administrator, not as an insurance company at risk for medical expenses. To confuse things further, many private insurance companies offer Medicare beneficiaries so-called wraparound policies to pay for what Medicare does not cover; when the intermediary and the wraparound policy company are the same, it becomes difficult to understand who is responsible for what.

The Federal Employees Health Benefit Program (FEHBP) is a unique government program. Under this program, the federal government acts as an employer and makes health insurance plans or MCOs available to federal employees. Thus, the federal government is acting like any other employer in this regard. Consequently, the FEHBP is best understood not as a government program but as an employer-based group health benefits plan.

Insurance

People purchase health care insurance to protect themselves from unexpected medical costs. The insurer provides coverage of medical costs at a premium rate that is calculated to cover those costs on average. To differentiate health care insurance from government health benefits plans, insurance is often referred to as "commercial" insurance (or "commercial" managed care in the case of an MCO).

The central point of health insurance is that the risk for medical expenses belongs to the insurance company. In other words, in exchange for the payment of insurance premiums, which can vary considerably in amount, the insurance company assumes the responsibility for paying the cost of medical benefits provided to individuals—that is, the cost of those benefits covered by the insurance policy in the first place. Other than the cost of the premium, as well as any applicable copayments (a fixed amount paid by the patient for each service), coinsurance (a percentage of cost for service paid by the insurance company with remaining percentage paid by patient), and/or deductible (a set amount of money that the patient must pay before any coverage is available), an insured individual is not at risk for the cost of medical care covered by the insurance policy. However, all insurance or managed care policies exclude certain medical care, such as experimental treatments or other care that is considered unnecessary. In other cases, there may be limits on what is covered—for example, a limit on the number of mental health visits per year.

With the notable exceptions of the Health Insurance Portability and Accountability Act (HIPAA) and, to a lesser degree, ERISA, the federal government does not regulate the insurance industry. Rather, regulation of the industry is the responsibility of the state governments. The regulatory system is highly complex and is discussed in greater detail in Chapter 7.

Each state taxes insurance via a premium tax; in other words, a small percentage of the premium charged to the purchaser is actually a tax. Most states have also passed mandated benefits laws that require insurance policies to provide coverage for defined diseases, providers, procedures, and so forth, but these vary from state to state. The states also have different laws and regulations regarding how health plans contract with providers, as well as the manner in which insurance is actually sold, to ensure that each sale is fair and that the terms of coverage are fully disclosed.

They also have different laws and regulations regarding how and when certain types of premiums may be charged to particular types of consumers or employers. These are important issues because the medical expenses of everyone in the coverage "pool" affect the insurance premium rates. In other words, if one employer group has high medical costs, the premium rates for all the other employer groups go up as well. The degree of that effect is determined by the type of policy.

Finally, it is common for insurance companies and MCOs, especially small to mid-sized health plans, to insure themselves against catastrophic costs. In other words, if the medical costs of any individuals or groups covered by the health plan become exceedingly high, the health plan has a reinsurance policy to cover some of the risk. This reinsurance policy "insures the insurer." Large insurance companies and MCOs may not always need reinsurance policies because they have large financial reserves and can absorb changes in medical costs.

Group Health Benefits Plans

Employers generally purchase insurance policies to provide group health benefit plans for their eligible employees, though not all employers offer insurance. Even when an employer does offer health insurance, not all employees may be considered eligible, however; in fact, temporary or part-time employees are seldom eligible to participate in an employer's health insurance benefits plan.

Group health benefits plans have several advantages:

- The cost of the insurance is paid on a pretax basis.
- Employers, especially large employers, are usually able to obtain more favorable pricing and coverage than individuals can.

- Health insurance benefits may be combined with other types of benefits (e.g., flexible spending accounts, health reimbursement accounts, or life insurance).
- The employer, not the individual employee, manages administrative needs such as payroll deductions, payment of premiums, and so forth.

The most common type of group health benefits plan is the defined benefits insurance plan. In this type of plan, the benefits offered in the insurance policy are defined by what the employer has purchased on behalf of the employees. It is common for an employer to offer more than one type of defined benefits plan, however. For example, an employee may be able to choose (at different cost to the employee, of course) between a high-option insurance plan, a low-option insurance plan (i.e., with lesser levels of coverage), a managed care plan with more restrictions but higher benefits and lower costs, and so forth. The larger the employer is, the more likely that multiple health plans will be available to the employees.

If premium costs for a group health benefits plan increase, as they usually do each year, the employer generally absorbs much of that cost increase. The employees commonly must also contribute part of their pretax earnings toward the cost of the insurance, usually around 25 percent of the cost of the insurance. This means that as insurance costs rise, the amount that an employee contributes may be the same on a percentage basis but will still be a higher absolute dollar amount. An employer may set that payroll deduction (i.e., the amount that the employee must pay) to favor lower cost choices; for example, there may be a lower payroll deduction if the employee chooses a lower cost plan. In all cases, however, the payroll deduction is pretax, meaning that it is not considered income for purposes of calculating the employee's income tax.

Wraparound, or Supplemental Health Insurance

An insurance policy that covers what another insurance policy or Medicare does not cover is called a wraparound, or supplemental insurance, policy. For example, a group health benefits plan may have a high deductible and a lifetime limit on certain costs. It may even exclude coverage for certain conditions. A wraparound policy would provide the missing coverage, subject to its own limitations. Wraparound policies in the commercial insurance sector are less common than they once were.

The most common type of wraparound insurance policies are those that are sold to Medicare beneficiaries. Because Medicare has relatively high deductibles and coinsurance and limits or does not cover all types of services, a wraparound policy is designed to cover those costs, though the degree of coverage varies with

different types of policies. Medicare wraparound policies must comply with requirements defined by CMS. With the advent of the new Medicare prescription
drug benefit and Medicare Advantage (see Chapter 6), such wraparound policies
have become less attractive to Medicare beneficiaries who now have more available options.

Individual Health Insurance

Individuals may be able to purchase health insurance policies directly from commercial insurance companies. In general, individual health insurance policies are
far more expensive and provide far less coverage than group policies. Exceptions
are policies that are sold to young and healthy individuals, though changes in laws
and regulations in many states have placed some limitations on how the premiums for young and healthy individuals may differ from those for older and sicker
individuals. In many cases, unless they can meet certain strict criteria, individuals with existing medical problems may not even be able to buy health insurance.

Some states do have laws requiring an "insurer of last resort," almost always a
not-for-profit health plan, to provide so-called guaranteed issue policies to anybody
who applies for one during a defined period each year. Such policies are always very
expensive and have limits on coverage. A few states have "catastrophic risk pools"
in which all insurers are required to contribute, with the funds being used to help
subsidize health insurance for individuals with significant medical problems.

Individuals who lose their jobs for any reason also lose their eligibility for the
group health benefits plan offered by their former employer. Under the Consolidated Omnibus Reconciliation Act (COBRA), as discussed further in Chapter 7,
they are eligible to maintain their participation in the group policy at a small increase in cost over the group premium rate for up to 18 months, but only if they
comply with strict requirements about when they apply for the COBRA extension and pay their premiums in a timely way. Under HIPAA, they may also be eligible to purchase individual health insurance policies by meeting strict criteria,
but the cost of such policies is usually quite high. Laws and regulations surrounding individual health insurance are highly complex and may differ from
those surrounding group health benefits plans. Suffice it to say that individual
health insurance is usually the least favorable option open to most consumers,
short of no insurance at all.

Finally, at the time that this book is being revised, several states have begun to
experiment with ways to broaden access to health insurance for those who lack it.

Health insurance market reform is also the subject of renewed political debate at the federal level, though no clear direction has as yet emerged.

Self-Funded Health Benefits Plans

Most large corporations do not actually insure their employees at all in the sense that they do not actually purchase health insurance from an insurance company. They escape the burdens of purchasing insurance through self-funding as allowed by ERISA. Assuming the risk of medical costs makes it possible for a large employer to avoid paying state premium tax and offering state-mandated benefits; furthermore, the costs of its own group (its employees and their dependents) alone determine its costs. Self-funded benefits plans are not regulated by the states in any way, but they are regulated by the U.S. Department of Labor. As a practical matter, as long as an employer complies with the requirements under ERISA, there is very little regulation involved.

It is most common for a large employer to contract with a third-party administrator to perform the management activities required by the self-funded health benefits plan. Often, the third-party administrator is actually a large insurance company or a Blue Cross Blue Shield plan, thus confusing both members and providers as to who the insurer actually is. These large insurance companies provide not only administrative services but also substantial discounts to the employers when they receive such discounts from the providers. Self-funded plans may mimic any type of insurance coverage.

Almost every employer with a self-funded health benefits plan purchases reinsurance to protect itself from extraordinarily high medical costs. In other words, the self-funded plan actually does have some level of insurance, though it is very high-level insurance and only for very high costs. If the third-party administrator managing the self-funded health benefits plan is a very large insurance company, a Blue Cross Blue Shield plan, or an MCO, the third-party administrator itself may provide the reinsurance. If the third-party administrator is small or is not a large insurer in its own right, then the employer must purchase reinsurance directly. Most states have rules regarding how much reinsurance a self-funded health benefits plan can have before it is considered an actual commercial group health insurance plan and therefore subject to state regulation; for example, if an employer purchases reinsurance to cover expenses that are only 5 percent higher than what was budgeted for, the state will claim that the employer is not self-funded and has actually purchased insurance, and therefore must comply with all state laws and regulations.

PAYER-BASED MANAGED CARE

As noted earlier, serious challenges are associated with attempting to describe the types of organizations in a field as dynamic as managed care. The health care system in the United States has been continually evolving, and change is the only constant. Nevertheless, distinctions remain between different MCOs, though many of those distinctions are rooted in the historic classifications that separated different forms of managed care, particularly during its time of rapid growth (see Chapter 1).

Originally, HMOs, PPOs, and traditional forms of indemnity health insurance were distinct, mutually exclusive products and mechanisms for providing health care coverage. Today, an observer may be hard pressed to uncover the differences among products that bill themselves as HMOs, PPOs, or managed care overlays to health insurance. The advent of CDHPs in the early part of the 2000s does provide a greater difference when compared with other types of health plans (and these will be discussed later in this chapter), though many aspects of managed health care are found in such plans.

For other types of health plans (i.e., non-CDHPs), differences in plan type may be hard to distinguish. For example, many HMOs, which traditionally limited their members to a designated set of participating providers, now allow their members to use nonparticipating providers at a reduced coverage level. Such POS plans combine HMO-like systems with indemnity systems, allowing individual members to choose which systems they wish to access at the time they need the medical service. POS rose and fell in popularity as a plan design, however, and is no longer as prevalent as it once was. Many PPOs, although not implementing a primary care physician (PCP) case management system, often provide for lower copayments by members to see a PCP and require higher copayments to see a specialty physician, thus encouraging a de facto form of PCP care management. Finally, almost all indemnity insurance (or self-insurance) plans now include utilization management (UM) features and provider networks in their plans, which were once found only in HMOs or PPOs (though indemnity insurance is now a quite rare form of coverage in any event).

As a result of these changes, the descriptions of the different types of managed care systems that follow provide only a guideline for determining the form of MCO that is observed. In many cases (or in most cases in some markets), the MCO will be a hybrid of several specific types.

Further confusing this is the existence of IDSs. In the never-ending quest to label different types of MCOs, which has all the stability of Jell-O® in an earthquake, some of these types of IDSs even require licensure from the state if they accept risk for medical costs—for example, a limited Knox-Keene license in California. IDSs are further discussed later in this chapter.

CDHPs, which combine a high-deductible insurance policy with a PPO network and a unique pretax "up-front" financing mechanism, do not fit neatly on the continuum as described next, however. Because of this, and their continued rapid evolution, they are described later in the chapter, separate from the more traditional types of managed care plans.

The Continuum of Managed Care

Managed care may be thought of as a continuum of models (Figure 2–2). These models are generally classified as follows:

- Indemnity with precertification, mandatory second opinion, and case management
- Service plan with precertification, mandatory second opinion, and case management
- Preferred provider organization (PPO)
- Point-of-service (POS) health plan
- "Open-access" HMO
- Traditional HMO
    1. Open-panel HMO
        –Independent practice association (IPA)
        –Direct contract HMO
    2. Network model
    3. Closed-panel HMO
        –Group model
        –Staff model

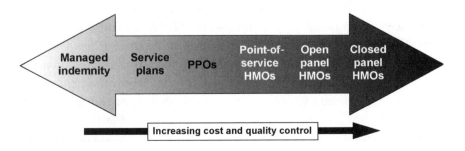

FIGURE 2–2 Continuum of Managed Care

As models move toward the managed care end of the continuum, the following features begin to appear:

- Tighter elements of control over health care delivery
- Addition of new elements of control
- More direct interaction with providers
- Increased overhead cost and complexity
- Greater control of utilization
- Net reduction in rate of rise of medical costs

Although it would be comforting to classify all MCOs using the above models, MCOs are anything but uniform and rarely occur in a pure form.

The classification of health plans that follows has little to do with who carries the actual risk for medical expenses, which was the basis of the discussion of risk bearing entities earlier in the chapter. The same terms may be used, but their meaning is different here. For instance, the terms "traditional insurance plan" and "service plan" now apply to certain kinds of health plans because of the structure and functioning of these plans, not their assumption of risk. To carry the example further, a traditional insurance plan may be either a truly traditional insurance plan in which the insurance company bears the risk for medical costs, or a self-funded health benefits plan in which the employer bears the risk; from the viewpoint of a member or a provider, however, there is no difference.

Finally, although various forms of reimbursement and medical management approaches will be mentioned, they will not be fully described here, but in Chapters 3 and 4.

Traditional Health Insurance

Basically, there are two types of traditional health insurance: indemnity insurance and service plans. It is called traditional because it used to be the dominant form of coverage, not because it still is. The costs of traditional health insurance rose rapidly beginning in the early to mid-1970s, becoming very expensive compared with costs of other types of managed care plans. As their costs rose, traditional insurers imposed ever-increasing cost sharing with the consumer, attempting to slow down cost increases. But employers moved away from traditional health insurance and into types of coverage that had larger elements of managed care. Traditional insurance has now shrunk to occupy only a tiny fraction of the market for health care coverage.

Indemnity Insurance

Indemnity insurance protects (indemnifies) the insured (i.e., the consumer or patient) against financial losses from medical expenses. The only restrictions are in the schedule of benefits listed in the insurance policy (i.e., what is covered by the policy). There are generally no restrictions on the licensed providers from whom the insured can seek care. The insurance company reimburses the subscriber directly for medical expenses, or it may pay the provider directly, although it has no actual obligation other than to pay the subscriber. Payment to physicians and other professional providers is subject to usual, customary, or reasonable (UCR) fee screens, whereas payment to institutional providers is generally based on charges.

Benefits are generally subject to a deductible (a flat dollar amount that the subscriber must pay before the insurance company pays anything) and coinsurance (a percentage of the covered charge that the subscriber pays, such as 20 percent). Any charges by the provider that the insurance company does not pay are strictly the responsibility of the subscriber.

Most indemnity plans require precertification of elective hospital admissions and may apply a financial penalty to the subscriber who fails to obtain precertification. The plan may also require some additional utilization management of hospital cases, but plan-employed nurses working at a remote site generally take care of utilization issues over the telephone. Case management may also be used to help control the cost of catastrophic cases in which costs are very high (e.g., a severely premature infant, or trauma cases). Second opinions may also be mandatory for certain elective procedures (e.g., surgery for obesity).

Service Plans

The term service plan applies primarily, though not exclusively, to Blue Cross and Blue Shield plans. In service plans, there are generally few restrictions on licensed providers who agree to sign a contract with the plan. The provider contract contains certain key provisions:

- The plan agrees to reimburse the provider directly, eliminating collection problems with patients.
- The provider agrees to accept the plan's fee schedule as payment in full and not to bill the subscriber for any payment not made by the plan (other than the normal deductible and coinsurance).
- The provider agrees to allow the plan to audit the provider's records.

Like indemnity insurance, service plans may require precertification, case management, and second opinions.

The principal advantage of a service plan over indemnity insurance is in the provider contracts and the reimbursement models that the contracts support. Professional fees allowed under the fee schedule represent a discount to the plan. More important, the plan usually has significant discounts at hospitals that give it a competitive advantage. The hospitals grant these discounts for a variety of reasons, including large volume of business, rapid payment, ease of collection, and, occasionally, advance deposits. The actual reimbursement to the hospital may be based on charges, diagnosis-related groups (DRGs), or some variation.

Preferred Provider Organizations

Although PPOs are similar to service plans, there are some important differences. A PPO may reduce the total panel of providers to some degree, sometimes substantially (e.g., 30 percent of the total number of providers available in the area). There are two broad approaches that a PPO may take to establish a panel: "any willing provider" acceptance versus criteria-based selection. In the former, any provider who wishes to participate in the organization and who agrees to the terms and conditions of the PPO's contract must be offered a contract, at least until the PPO has adequate numbers of providers. In the latter, the PPO uses some objective criteria (e.g., credentials, practice pattern analysis) that a provider must meet before receiving a contract offer. Any willing provider PPOs are more common, particularly following numerous state laws requiring it, but the use of criteria-based selection still occurs, particularly with expensive or highly specialized services (e.g., for cardiac surgery).

Although PPO payment mechanisms to providers may fall along the lines mentioned under service plans, the discounts are generally greater. Many service plans require providers to give them "most favored nation" pricing; in other words, a provider may not offer a better discount to a competitor than it does to the service plan. Such favored-nation pricing has become less common recently because of regulatory and legal pressure, and it is even prohibited in a number of states.

Precertification and case management are almost always components of PPOs (mandatory second opinion programs are relatively uncommon because they are no longer considered to be effective). The main difference between a PPO and a traditional health insurance plan is that failure to comply with these programs results in a financial penalty to the provider, not the subscriber. As with service plans, a contracting provider may not bill the subscriber for any balance that the

PPO does not pay, except for the normal deductible and coinsurance. In the event that a subscriber chooses to seek care from a nonparticipating provider, the responsibility falls on the subscriber, and the subscriber is at risk for any charges not paid by the PPO.

A hallmark of a PPO is that benefits are reduced if a member seeks care from a provider who is not in the PPO network. A common benefits differential is 20 percent. For example, if a member sees a network provider, coverage is provided at 80 percent of allowed charges; if a member sees a provider not in the network, the coverage may be at the 60 percent level.

PPOs can be either risk bearing or non-risk bearing. A risk-bearing PPO combines the insurance, or payment, function with the management of the network of providers. A non-risk-bearing PPO focuses solely on network management, not on the insurance function. For example, a commercial insurer may build a network and sell coverage to clients; this insurer is a risk-bearing PPO. Alternatively, a group of providers may come together as a legal entity, establish professional principles (e.g., fee allowances, credentialing criteria, utilization review), and contract with independent insurers to provide medical services to those insurers' customers; this organization is a non-risk-bearing PPO. Non-risk-bearing PPOs that contract with multiple insurers are also referred to as rental PPOs.

PPOs are far less expensive than traditional insurance, though usually more expensive than HMOs unless the PPO has a high degree of cost sharing with consumers. Because of the issues around the managed care backlash (discussed in Chapter 1), PPOs have the largest share of the market.

Point-of-Service Plans

POS plans combine features of HMOs and traditional insurance plans. In a POS plan, members may choose which system to use at the point at which they obtain the service. For example, if a member uses his or her PCP and otherwise complies with the HMO authorization system, the benefits for services may be quite generous, and the member would be required to pay only a minor copayment. If the member chooses to self-refer or otherwise not to use the HMO system to receive services, the plan still provides insurance coverage but would require a higher deductible and higher coinsurance. The difference between coverage for in-network services and out-of-network services generally ranges from 20 percent to 40 percent.

Point-of-service plans developed because of the conflict between cost control and total freedom of choice of providers. By bringing the issue of cost differential directly to HMO members at the point at which they seek medical services, the members would be more active participants in the process. Initially popular, they have become less common in recent years because their cost has not been favorable when compared with either PPOs (with more cost sharing) or HMOs (with more controls).

Health Maintenance Organizations

HMOs are fundamentally different from the health plans just described. Although there are exceptions, known as "open-access" HMOs, that are similar in benefits design to PPOs, the majority of HMOs manage utilization and quality to a greater degree than do PPOs. With some exceptions, benefits to members in an HMO must be provided by the HMO's providers in compliance with the HMO's authorization procedures. Benefits obtained through the HMO are almost always significantly more generous than those found in any other type of health plan. Except in true emergencies or specifically authorized instances, payment for services received from non-HMO providers is the responsibility of the subscriber, not the HMO. Services delivered by contracted providers who fail to obtain proper authorization are the responsibility of the provider, who may not bill the subscriber for any fees not paid by the HMO.

Traditional HMOs currently fall into two broad categories: open panel and closed panel. A third category, the true network model, is relatively uncommon except in certain parts of the country. Some HMOs combine or mix different model types in the same market. Because open-access HMOs are not considered traditional HMOs, they are discussed separately, followed by a discussion of traditional open- and closed-panel plans.

Open-Access HMOs

Open-access HMOs are more like PPOs than traditional HMOs. In the open-access HMO model, members may access any provider in the HMO without going through a PCP. Thus, members may see any PCP or specialist in the network on a self-referral basis. The physicians in the open-access HMO share at least some level of risk for costs. Therefore, if professional costs exceed the budget, the physicians may have to accept lower fees, lose their withhold (i.e., the amount of payment that the HMO holds back to cover higher-than-budgeted medical costs) if those are being used, and so forth.

Open-access plans were popular in the late 1970s and early 1980s, especially plans sponsored by organized medical societies. With a few exceptions, these early plans suffered substantial losses and failed. A revival of interest in open-access plans occurred, however, because of consumer demands. Such demands are certainly logical: Who does not want a health care plan with a high level of benefits, low costs, and unlimited access to providers? The HMOs that are currently using an open-access design are doing so on the assumption that, because so few referral authorizations are denied, the referral requirement is not worth the cost. However, a PCP will be able to deliver routine care more cost-effectively than a specialist. Therefore, most open-access HMOs have substantial cost-sharing differences for care provided by a specialist compared with that provided by a PCP. Most open-access HMOs also provide substantially lower benefits or no benefits at all for nonemergency care received from nonnetwork providers.

Open-Panel Plans

In an open-panel HMO, private physicians and other professional providers are independent contractors who see HMO members in their own offices. They may contract with more than one competing health plan (and usually do) and also see fee-for-service patients. A variety of reimbursement mechanisms may be used. The total number of providers in an open-panel plan is larger than that in a closed-panel plan but usually smaller than in a PPO. Each member must choose a single provider to be his or her PCP (sometimes referred to as a "gatekeeper"), who must authorize any other services. Members may change their PCPs at designated times if they wish.

Open-panel plans fall into two broad categories: independent practice associations (IPAs) and direct contract models. Although the terms are often used synonymously, the two models are technically distinct. In an IPA model, the HMO contracts with a legal entity known as an IPA (described later in this chapter) and pays it a negotiated capitation amount. The IPA, in turn, contracts with private physicians to provide health care to the HMO members. The IPA may pay the physicians through capitation or may use another mechanism, such as fee-for-service. The providers are at risk under this model in that if medical costs exceed the capitation amount, the IPA receives no additional funds from the HMO and must accordingly adjust its payments to the providers.

In the direct contract model, the HMO contracts directly with the providers; there is no intervening entity. The HMO pays the providers directly and performs all related management tasks. Direct contract HMOs are currently the most common type.

Open-panel HMOs are far more common than are closed panel plans.

Closed-Panel Plans

Unlike physicians in an open-panel plan, physicians in a closed-panel plan confine their practice to the HMO members. These physicians practice in facilities that are likewise dedicated to the HMO. The total number of providers in the closed-panel plan is by far the smallest of any model type. Members usually do not have to choose a single PCP but may see any PCP or any physician in the HMO facility; however, they may be asked to choose a primary facility to ensure continuity of care.

Closed-panel plans fall into two broad categories: group model and staff model. In a group model plan, the HMO contracts with a group of physicians to provide services to members. The HMO pays the group a negotiated capitation amount, and the group in turn pays the individual physicians through a combination of salary and risk/reward incentives. The group is responsible for its own governance, and the physicians are either partners in the group or associates. The group or the HMO may provide the dedicated practice facilities and support staff, but most commonly, the HMO assumes that responsibility. The group is at risk in that if the costs of the group exceed the capitation amount, the reimbursement to the providers is less—although the HMO generally provides stop-loss reinsurance to the group to protect the group from catastrophic cost overruns. Some groups exist primarily on paper and actually operate strictly as cost pass-through vehicles for the HMO (i.e., the costs are simply passed from the medical group to the HMO, and the group does not actually bear any risk for medical expenses); in this event, the arrangement resembles a staff model plan. The largest and best-known group model HMO is Kaiser Permanente.

In a staff model plan, the HMO contracts with the providers directly, and the providers are employees of the HMO. Physicians receive a salary, and there is an incentive plan of some sort. The HMO has full responsibility for the management of all activities. Staff model plans are almost extinct now.

Network Model HMOs

Occasionally, the term "network model" is used to refer to an open-panel plan, but in the "true" network model, the HMO contracts with several large multispecialty medical groups for services. The groups receive payment under capitation, and they in turn pay the physicians under a variety of mechanisms. The groups operate relatively independently. The HMO contracts with more than one group, but the number of groups is usually limited. True network models are most common in California.

Mixed-Model HMOs

Nothing in this world is pure and simple, and HMOs are no exception. Many HMOs have adopted several model types, even in the same market, to attract as many members as possible and capture additional market share. The most common form of mixed model involves grafting a direct contract model onto either a closed-panel or a network model. For example, the HMO may need to expand its medical service area and may choose to contract with private physicians rather than make the expenditures required for an additional facility. In mixed-model plans, the models often operate independently of each other.

Consumer-Directed Health Plans

CDHPs combine a high-deductible insurance plan with some form of pretax savings account. They are often associated with a PPO network as well. If there is no pretax savings feature, it may be referred to as a high-deductible health plan (HDHP). In a CDHP, health care costs are paid first from the pretax account, and when that is exhausted, any additional costs up to the deductible are paid out-of-pocket by the member (this gap is sometimes referred to as a bridge or a doughnut hole). Preventive services are usually covered outside of this system, however. The definition of preventive services varies among plans. Any funds left over in the savings account may roll over to be used in following years as needed.

There are two basic forms of CDHPs: commercial CDHPs that use health reimbursement accounts (HRAs), and plans associated with health savings accounts (HSAs). HSAs were created as part of the Medicare Modernization Act. They are a more rigid form of CDHP and include definitions of what constitutes preventive care and how high the deductible must be. HSAs are regulated by the U.S. Treasury Department. Commercial CDHPs with associated HRAs are also regulated by the U.S. Treasury Department, but that applies only to the HRA itself. HRA plan design is more flexible than HSAs, though subject to state insurance regulations or, in the case of self-funded business under ERISA, the U.S. Department of Labor. As a practical matter, the differences are not especially important to understanding the basics of CDHPs for purposes of this overview. An example of a simplistic schematic of a CDHP is illustrated in Figure 2-3.

CDHPs are not considered managed health care plans by some, who consider them as more akin to simpler indemnity-type insurance plans from the past. This is because of the presence of a high-deductible health insurance policy as the primary product, with new benefits in the form of preventive services combined with

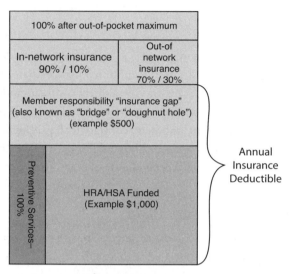

FIGURE 2–3 Example of Basic Construct of a Consumer-Directed Health Plan

new pretax funding mechanisms for at least a portion of the costs. But one of the primary arguments made by advocates of CDHPs is that the consumer has become shielded by managed care plans as to how much health really costs; in other words, consumers have come to believe that an office visit really only costs $20 or that a sophisticated diagnostic test only costs $40. The CDHP is therefore constructed to make cost a factor in consumer decision making through the use of both the pretax fund and the bridge, with the CDHP providing information to consumers to help them make decisions based on cost and quality of services.

CDHPs have not entirely shed all aspects of managed health care, however. Most are associated with a PPO to provide the value of the negotiated discount to the consumer. From the provider viewpoint, this is a mixed blessing because providers find that it is difficult to collect all the money owed to them when they must bill the consumer after the fact. Integrating the functions of the HRAs or HSAs through debit cards and finding ways for the provider to collect what is due at the time of service is a major focus of effort by insurance companies offering CDHPs.

Simply integrating with an existing PPO is the most common, but not the only, aspect of managed care that CDHPs retain. Integration of medical management into the new plan designs is still evolving, particularly with CDHPs offered by the larger and more established companies. Disease management (DM) and case management (CM), both discussed in Chapter 4, are most frequently applied because a only a small percentage of people account for a high percentage of medical costs. But how a CDHP applies DM in the early stages of a chronic disease is still evolving.

INTEGRATED DELIVERY SYSTEMS

Like MCOs, organized health care delivery systems, known as IDSs, fall into various categories. Most IDSs* have been established to make it easier for different types of providers to work together in a managed care environment. IDSs contract with MCOs, coordinate the care delivered to patients, and enhance efficiencies in the health care delivery system overall. The success of IDSs in meeting these goals has been mixed, and many large IDSs have failed in the past. Other IDSs have achieved their goals, however, particularly the goals that are generally easier to achieve by larger organizations with correspondingly greater resources and negotiating leverage.

Like the classification system for MCOs, the classification system for IDSs is imprecise. Furthermore, the terms used to describe IDSs rival those in the rest of the managed care industry for sheer number and vagueness of definition. Following is a list of names and acronyms for some of the main types of IDSs:

- Independent practice association (IPA)
- Physician-hospital organization (PHO)
- Management services organization (MSO)
- Provider-sponsored organization (PSO)
- Physician practice management company (PPMC)
- Group practice without walls (GPWW)
- Medical group practice
- Foundation model
- Staff model

Multiple IDSs may exist within any single health care delivery system, and the definition and actual activities of an IDS may not be the same from one organization to another. For example, an IDS may contain an IPA to organize independent physicians, a PPMC to manage the physician practices owned by the

---

* Some legal and tax professionals prefer to reserve the term "integrated delivery system" for distinct corporate entities that operate under a single identity for purposes of taxation and liability. This book makes no such distinction.

hospital, a PHO to serve as the contracting vehicle for the IDS's contracts with MCOs, and so forth. The following is a brief description of the most common types of IDSs or components of IDSs.

Independent Practice Association

IPAs have been in existence for several decades. Members of an IPA are independent physicians who contract with the IPA, which is a legal entity, so that the IPA can contract with one or more MCOs. Although most IPAs are nonprofit, some are for-profit. The term "independent practice association" is commonly used to refer to any type of open-panel HMO, but this usage is not technically correct. Usually, an IPA is an umbrella organization for physicians in all specialties to participate in managed care. However, IPAs representing only a single specialty also exist.

In a typical case, the IPA negotiates with an HMO for a capitation rate that takes into account all physician services. The IPA, in turn, pays the member physicians, although not necessarily according to a capitation rate; in fact, many pay physicians on a fee-for-service basis. The IPA and its member physicians are at risk for at least some portion of medical costs in that if the capitation rate is too low to cover the physician payments, the physicians must accept a lower income. It is the presence of this risk sharing that distinguishes the IPA from a negotiating vehicle that does not bear risk. It is also the reason that a true IPA is not typically subject to antitrust lawsuits (unless it was formed solely or primarily to keep out competition). It is a problem for IPAs to negotiate with PPOs around fee schedules, because that may be considered illegal price fixing and antitrust in the absence of risk sharing. The IPA generally has stop-loss reinsurance (or is provided such insurance by the HMO) to avoid going bankrupt.

An IPA may operate simply as a negotiating organization, with the HMO providing all administrative support, or it may take on some of the duties of the HMO, such as utilization management or network development. In some cases, particularly if the IPA is large and mature, the IPA may also adjudicate claims.

Physician-Hospital Organization

By definition, a PHO requires the participation of a hospital and at least some portion of the admitting physicians. At a minimum, a PHO is an entity that allows a hospital and its affiliated physicians to negotiate with MCOs. In its weakest form, it operates solely as a messenger: the PHO analyzes the terms and conditions offered by an MCO and transmits the analysis and the contract to each physician, who then decides on an individual basis whether to participate. It is not uncommon for the same physicians who join a PHO to already be under contract with one or more managed care plans.

Typically, the participating physicians and the hospital develop model contract terms and reimbursement levels and use those to negotiate with MCOs. The PHO usually has a limited amount of time to negotiate a contract successfully (e.g., 90 days). If the time limit passes without an agreement, then the participating physicians are free to contract directly with the MCO. If the PHO successfully reaches an agreement with the MCO, then the physicians agree to be bound by the terms of the PHO's contract with the MCO. Confusingly, the actual contract for health care services is still between the physician and the MCO or between the hospital and the MCO. In some cases, the contract between the physicians and the MCO is relatively concise and may refer to the contract between the PHO and the MCO.

A PHO may actively manage the relationship between the providers and MCOs. It is usually a separate business entity, such as a for-profit corporation. How equity or ownership is divided between the physicians and the hospital, where the money comes from to operate the PHO, and how (or even if) money comes into the PHO from its managed care activities are all complex issues that must be resolved. One last note regarding PHOs: The physician portion of a PHO may itself be a different type of IDS, such as an IPA, and there are other methods of organization as well.

Management Services Organization

An MSO differs from a PHO in that not only does the MSO provide a vehicle for negotiating with MCOs, but it also offers additional services to support the physicians' practices. The physicians, however, usually remain independent private practitioners. An MSO is based around one or more hospitals. The reasons for an MSO's formation are generally the same as those for the formation of a PHO (primarily contract negotiation), and the ownership and operational issues are similar.

In its simplest form, an MSO operates as a service bureau, providing basic practice support services to member physicians. These services often include billing and collection, administrative support in certain areas, and electronic data interchange. The physicians can remain independent practitioners, under no legal obligation to use the services of the hospital on an exclusive basis. The MSO must receive payment from the physicians at fair market value for the services that the MSO does provide, however, or the hospital and the physicians could incur legal problems.

Some MSOs may be considerably broader in scope. In addition to providing all the services that have been described, an MSO may actually purchase many of the assets of a physician's practice. For example, the MSO may purchase the physician's office space or office equipment (at fair market value), can employ the office support staff of the physician, and can even perform functions such as quality management, utilization management, provider relations, member services, and claims processing. An MSO of this type is usually constructed as a unique business entity separate from a PHO.

An MSO does not always directly contract with MCOs for two reasons. First, many MCOs insist that the providers themselves be the contracting agents (to be sure that the providers understand and agree to the contractual terms and to make sure that the contract remains in force even if the MSO ceases to exist). Second, many states will not allow MCOs (especially HMOs) to have contracts with any entity that does not have the power to bind the provider—something that an MSO may not be able to do because the physicians may remain independent private practitioners, and as independent providers, they could refuse to honor contract terms that they themselves did not sign.

Provider-Sponsored Organization

Generally, a PSO is a cooperative venture of a group of providers who control the venture's health service delivery and financial arrangements. In effect, a PSO is an integrated provider system engaged in both delivering and financing health care services. Its focus is typically on the Medicare population, but it could theoretically expand to include commercial and Medicaid initiatives as well.

The Balanced Budget Act of 1997 provided for the creation of PSOs to provide a vehicle that would allow providers to contract directly with Medicare to accept risk for services and costs to an enrolled group of Medicare beneficiaries. The act required the PSO to provide a substantial portion of health care directly or through affiliated groups of providers and for the providers themselves to have at least a majority ownership interest in the PSO. In an urban area, a substantial portion of health care services is defined as 70 percent or more (as measured by expenditures); in a rural area, it is defined as 60 percent or more.

When the act created PSOs, there was a general belief that they would eliminate the administrative overhead costs associated with Medicare HMOs and that providers themselves would be better positioned to manage both the cost and the quality of health care for Medicare beneficiaries. These assumptions proved to be false, and almost all PSOs that came into existence failed within a few years, often experiencing spectacular losses and creating substantial managerial pain within the provider systems themselves. A few PSOs succeeded however, and still exist.

Physician Practice Management Company

In the early to mid-1990s, PPMCs arrived on the scene, and they acquired physician practices throughout the middle to late 1990s. PPMCs may be viewed as variant MSOs, but unlike the MSOs described earlier, PPMCs are for physicians only. In other words, hospitals have no involvement. Some authorities refer to these organizations as physician-only MSOs. A PPMC could be inclusive of many specialties or be focused on a single specialty (e.g., cardiology).

In general, a PPMC manages all support functions (e.g., billing and collections, purchasing, contract negotiations) but remains relatively uninvolved with the clinical aspects of a physician's practice. In many cases, the physician remains an independent practitioner, although the PPMC owns all the tangible assets of the practice. The PPMC usually takes a percentage of the practice revenue, often at a rate equal to or slightly below the physician's previous overhead costs. The physician makes a long-term commitment to the PPMC and agrees not to compete with the other physicians if he or she leaves the company.

It was hoped that PPMCs, usually organized on a for-profit basis, would achieve more efficient management and economies of scale, thereby producing a profit while maintaining physician income. Practice acquisitions were expected to give PPMCs a stronger negotiating position with MCOs, at least when a PPMC represented a substantial percentage of the physicians in a given area. Many PPMCs also sought global capitation contracts (i.e., contracts covering administrative and medical services), and in general, they desired to cut out the hospital from any profit and control.

Some practitioners, exasperated by the pressures of running a practice, preferred selling their practices to a PPMC rather than a hospital, possibly because they distrusted the hospital or expected the PPMC to have greater practice management capability. Unfortunately, in most cases, these physicians were severely disappointed. Not only did the PPMCs fail to demonstrate the management expertise that the physicians expected, but the practice acquisitions made the physicians into employees (or employee-like staff members) for many years. The physicians, having received a substantial payment for selling their practice as well as a guaranteed salary, had little incentive to work hard.

In general, the track record of PPMCs is terrible, and they fell to ruin in large numbers. Most major PPMCs have disappeared, either through bankruptcy or by exiting the business. Because some PPMCs are doing well, particularly single-specialty PPMCs, it is not appropriate to dismiss the concept out of hand, but currently they are not a significant type of IDS.

Group Practice without Walls

Also known as the clinic without walls, the GPWW is a step toward greater integration of small physician practices. It does not require the participation of a hospital and indeed is often the result of physicians' desire to organize without being dependent on a hospital for services or support. In some cases, GPWW formation has occurred to take advantage of the strength that numbers give in negotiating with MCOs and with hospitals.

A GPWW is composed of private practice physicians who agree to combine their practices into a single legal entity but continue to practice medicine in their independent locations. In other words, the physicians appear to be independent from the point of view of their patients, but they are a single group from the point of view of a contracting entity (usually an MCO). Two features differentiate GPWWs from PPMCs: First, the GPWW is owned solely by the member physicians and not by any outside investors, and second, the GPWW is a legal merging of all assets of the physician practices rather than the acquisition of only the tangible assets (as is often the case in a PPMC).

The member physicians own and govern the GPWW. They may contract with an outside organization for business support services. Office support services are generally provided through the group, although the physicians may notice little difference in their day-to-day office procedures.

For various legal and organizational reasons, the GPWW is a model that has not become common, much less dominant. Many state and federal enforcement agencies have concluded that without significant sharing of operations and financial risk, some GPWWs existed solely for anticompetitive price negotiating, causing the GPWW to either become a real group practice or to dissolve. Because they do accept risk from HMOs, they have done well in California.

Medical Group Practice

Traditionally, physicians who have wanted to combine their resources have done so in truly unified medical group practices. Unlike the GPWW, in which the physicians combine certain assets and risks but continue to practice medicine in their own offices, the true medical group has one or a small number of locations and functions as a group. That is, there is a great deal of interaction among the members of the group, as well as common goals and objectives. Traditional medical groups are legally independent of hospitals. Even so, it is common for a group to identify strongly with one hospital or health system. A number of traditional medical groups formed group model HMOs, though most of those evolved into mixed models to grow.

A medical group is usually a partnership or professional corporation, although other forms are possible. Usually, the more senior members of the group enjoy more of the fruits of the group's success (e.g., higher income, better on-call schedules). An existing group often requires new members to complete a probationary period and to make a substantial contribution to the group's capital upon joining, which can create an entry barrier and slow growth. Other groups simply employ new physicians for a lengthy period in order to control the finances of the group (new physicians are paid considerably less than senior physicians) and to give all parties the opportunity to see whether they can work together successfully. In any event, it is common for a medical group to require a noncompete clause in each physician's contract to protect the group from physician defections and the taking away of patients.

In a medical group, the performance of the group as a whole affects the personal income of the member physicians. Although an IPA places a defined portion of a physician's income at risk (that portion related to the managed care contract held by the IPA), the medical group's income from any source determines the individual physician's income and profit; that being said, an individual physician's productivity is commonly the most important factor in determining his or her income while part of a medical group.

Foundation Model

In one type of foundation model IDS, a hospital creates a nonprofit foundation and actually purchases physician practices (both tangible and intangible assets) and puts those practices into the foundation. This model is often used when a hospital cannot employ the physicians directly or use hospital funds to purchase the practices directly (as might be the case if the hospital is a nonprofit entity that cannot own a for-profit subsidiary, or if a state law prohibits the corporate practice of medicine). To qualify for and maintain its nonprofit status, the foundation must prove that it provides substantial benefits to the community.

A second form of foundation model does not involve a hospital. In that model, the foundation is an independent entity that contracts for services with a medical group and a hospital. On a historical note, in the early days of HMOs, many open-panel plans that were not formed as IPAs were formed as foundations; the foundation held the HMO license and contracted with one or more IPAs and hospitals for services.

The foundation itself is governed by a board that is not dominated by either the hospital or the physicians (in fact, physician representation on the board is not allowed to be above 20 percent). The board includes lay members. The foundation owns and manages the practices, but the physicians become members of a medical group that in turn has an exclusive contract for services with the foundation; in other words, the foundation is the only source of revenue for the medical group. The physicians have long-term contracts with the medical group, and the contracts contain noncompete clauses.

Although the physicians are in an independent group and the foundation is independent of the hospital, the relationship between the three is close. The medical group, however, retains a significant measure of autonomy regarding its own business affairs, and the foundation has no control over certain aspects, such as individual physician compensation.

Staff Model

The distinction between the staff model associated with an HMO, as discussed earlier, and that associated with an IDS owned by a health system, is whether the principal business organization is a risk-bearing, licensed entity (e.g., an HMO) or primarily a provider. The staff model is a health system that employs the physicians directly. Physicians enter the system either through the purchase of their practices or through direct recruitment. The system usually comprises more than just a hospital; it is a large, comprehensive health care organization. Because the physicians are employees, the legal issues attached to IDSs using private physicians are reduced. Direct employment of physicians is not allowed in some states.

GOVERNANCE AND MANAGEMENT OF MCOs

The governance and management of an MCO is influenced by its type, its structure (or that of its parent company), and many other variables. The function of key officers or managers as well as of committees depends on the MCO's type, its ownership, and the motivations and skills of the individuals involved. Further, MCOs must comply with many legal and regulatory requirements (state and federal), and which requirements apply depends on the MCO's structure and features (e.g., whether it is for-profit or nonprofit, whether it is provider owned, its state of domicile, and what types of products it offers). Thus, each health care system must construct its own management control structure to suit its own needs.

Board of Directors

Many, but not all, managed care plans have a board of directors. Numerous factors influence the composition and function of the board, which has the final responsibility for the plan's operation. Plans that do not necessarily have their own boards include the following:

- PPOs developed by large insurance companies
- PPOs developed for single employers by an insurance company
- HMOs set up by a single company just for the purpose of serving the company's employees
- Employer-sponsored or employer-developed plans (PPOs, precertification operations)
- HMOs or exclusive provider organizations set up by an insurance company as a line of business

With one exception, each of these entities is a subsidiary of a larger company, and whereas the company does have a board of directors, the board oversees the entire company, not just the subsidiary. A PPO or HMO that is a division of an insurance company may be required to list a board on its licensure forms, but that board may have little real operational role. The one exception, as noted earlier, is an HMO set up by a single company to serve its employees; such an HMO is considered to be self-funded and is regulated by labor laws, not insurance laws.

Although most HMOs have boards of directors, not all those boards are completely functional. This is especially true for HMOs that are part of large national companies. Each local HMO is incorporated and required by law to have a board, but it is not uncommon for the national company to use the same corporate officers as the board for every local HMO. Though the board fulfills its legal function and obligation, control of the actual operation of the HMO comes through the management structure of the national company rather than through a direct relationship between the HMO executives and the board.

Membership

The composition of the board of directors varies depending on whether the plan is for-profit (in which case the owners' or shareholders' representatives may hold the majority of seats) or nonprofit (in which case community representation will be broader). Some nonprofit health plans are organized as cooperatives (i.e., a legal entity in which the members, or enrollees, are as a group in control of the entity), in which case the board members are all members of the plan. In nonprofit plans that are not cooperatives, board members generally should be truly independent and have no potential conflicts of interest; provider-sponsored nonprofit plans may restrict seats held by providers to no more than 20 percent. In any case, local events, company bylaws, and laws and regulations (including the tax code for nonprofit health plans) dictate whether the board members come from outside the health plan or from the staff of the plan. Because in a provider-sponsored for-profit plan the providers may have majority representation, they must take special precautions to avoid antitrust problems; for example, an objective outside party rather than the providers themselves must set fees.

Responsibilities

The function of an MCO board of directors is governance—overseeing the MCO's activities. Final approval of corporate bylaws rests with the board. It is the bylaws that determine the basic structure of power, both that of the plan officers and that of the board itself. Because significant liability issues surround the board of directors, each board member must undertake his or her duties with care and diligence.

The fiduciary responsibility of the board of directors (i.e., their duty to protect the organization's financial assets) is clear. The board's duties include not only general oversight of the MCO's profitability or reserve status (money in reserve for when costs exceed premium income) but also approval of significant fiscal events, such as a major acquisition or expenditure. In a for-profit plan, the board has fiduciary responsibility to protect the interests of the stockholders.

As part of their legal responsibilities, members of the board may have to review certain reports and sign particular documents. For example, a board officer may be required to sign the quarterly financial report to the state regulatory agency, and the board chairperson may be required to sign any acquisition documents. The board is also responsible for the veracity of financial statements sent to stockholders.

Policy making is another common function of an active board. This responsibility may be as broad as determining whether to use a gatekeeper system, or it may be as detailed as approving organization charts and reporting structures. Although the plan officers set most of the day-to-day policies and procedures, an active board may set a policy regarding what operational policies the officers must bring to the board for approval or change.

In HMOs and many other types of MCOs, the board of directors has special responsibilities in several areas. First is the oversight of the quality of care delivered to members, and the quality management program. Usually, the board carries out this responsibility through a review of the quality management documentation (including the overall quality management plan and regular reports on findings and activities), either by the full board or a board subcommittee, and through feedback to the medical director and plan quality management committee. Second is corporate compliance with privacy requirements under HIPAA and with Medicare requirements for those MCOs with Medicare contracts.

In freestanding plans, the board also has responsibility for hiring the chief executive officer (CEO) of the plan and for reviewing that officer's performance. The board in such plans often sets the CEO's compensation package, and the CEO reports to the board. The board of a publicly traded company also has increased financial oversight requirements, created by the Sarbanes-Oxley Act of 2002 in the wake of a number of financial scandals.

Active boards generally have committees for certain functions, including an executive committee (e.g., to make decisions rapidly), a compensation committee (e.g., to set general compensation guidelines for the plan's staff, set the CEO's compensation, and approve and issue stock options), a finance committee or audit committee (e.g., to review financial statistics, approve budgets, set and approve spending authority, review the annual audit, and review and approve outside funding sources), a corporate compliance committee, and a quality management committee.

Key Management Positions

The roles and titles of the key managers in any organization vary depending on the type of organization, its legal status, its line of business, its complexity, and whether it is a freestanding entity or a satellite of another operation, among other factors. There is little consistency from health plan to health plan. How each key role is defined (or even whether it is present at all) is strictly up to the management of each plan. Thus, it is possible to provide only a general overview of certain key roles (Figure 2–4).

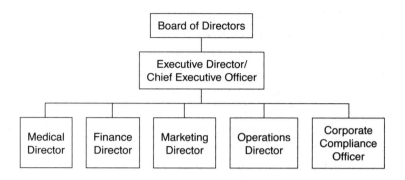

FIGURE 2–4 Key Management Positions in a Health Plan

Executive Director/Chief Executive Officer

Most plans have at least one key manager. Sometimes called an executive director, a CEO, a general manager, or a plan manager, this individual is usually responsible for all the operational aspects of the plan. This is not always the case, however. For example, some large companies (e.g., insurance companies or national HMO chains) have their local marketing directors report directly to a regional marketing director rather than to the local plan manager. A few companies take that to the extreme of having the chief of every functional area report to regional managers instead of to a single local manager. Thus, reporting is a function of the overall environment, and there is little standardization in the industry.

In freestanding plans and traditional HMOs, the CEO is responsible for all areas. The other officers and key managers report to the CEO, who in turn reports to the board (or to a regional manager in the case of national companies). The executive director also has responsibility for general administrative operations and public relations.

Medical Director/Chief Medical Officer

It can almost be assumed that managed care plans will have a medical director. The needs of the plan determine whether that position is full time or filled by a community physician who comes in a few hours a week, though such part-time involvement is becoming rare. The medical director usually has responsibility for provider relations, provider recruiting, quality management, utilization management, and medical policy. In large health plans and insurance companies, it is not uncommon for provider relations and network management to be independent of the medical director, however.

In some plans (e.g., simple PPOs), the medical director alone, or a medical consultant, may review claims, approve physician applications, and examine patterns of utilization. The intensity of medical director involvement parallels the level of medical management. Usually, the medical director reports to the executive director.

Finance Director/Chief Financial Officer

In freestanding plans or large operations, it is common to have a finance director or chief financial officer. That individual is generally responsible for all financial and accounting operations. In some plans, these operations include functions such as billing, enrollment, and underwriting (analyzing groups to determine rates and benefits), as well as accounting, fiscal reporting, and budget preparation. The person in this position usually reports to the executive director, although once again, some national companies require reporting to a higher level.

Marketing Director/Chief Marketing Officer

The responsibility for marketing the plan belongs to the marketing director. Responsibility generally includes oversight of marketing representatives, advertising, client relations, enrollment forecasting, and public relations. A few plans have the marketing department generate initial premium rates, which are then sent to the finance or underwriting department for review, but that is uncommon. The marketing director reports to the executive director or to someone at a higher level, depending on the company.

Operations Director/Chief Operating Officer

In larger plans, it is common to have an operations director or chief operating officer. It is also common in very large companies for this position to carry the title of president. The person in this position usually oversees claims, IT, enrollment, underwriting (unless finance is doing so), member services, office management, procurement, and any other traditional backroom functions. The operations director usually reports to the executive director.

Director of Information Services/Chief Information Officer

Information services have become sufficiently complex that all health plans have an officer dedicated to overseeing this function. Typical responsibilities include oversight of the data center (the physical computing equipment itself), all software and system applications, personal computer networks, telecommunications, Internet portals, and outsourced services. It is also common for this officer to oversee the maintenance of the physical offices of the company.

Corporate Compliance Officer

As mentioned previously, health plans have certain corporate compliance requirements. HIPAA contains extensive privacy requirements that an MCO must meet, and the MCO must appoint a specific individual responsible for ensuring that the organization is in compliance with these requirements. Similarly, an MCO with a Medicare Advantage contract needs a corporate compliance officer to ensure compliance with Medicare requirements. Finally, there are compliance requirements in the Sarbanes-Oxley Act. One corporate compliance officer may be able to fulfill all these responsibilities.

Other Common Positions

Depending on the size and complexity of a health plan or insurance company, there are numerous other positions that may exist. Functions such as legal affairs, strategic planning, investor relations, and the like routinely have their own dedicated executives. Large companies also tend to divide the responsibilities described earlier into many more senior level officers.

Committees

Again, there is little consistency from organization to organization regarding committees. Most organizations have nonmedical standing committees to address management issues in defined areas. In contrast, ad hoc committees, by definition, are convened to meet a specific need and then dissolved. A consumer or member advisory committee is a common type of nonmedical committee; although its members have no voting rights or governance powers, they provide consumer or member input to plan managers. In the medical management area, committees serve to diffuse some elements of responsibility (which can be beneficial for medical-legal reasons) and allow important input from providers into procedures and policies or even into case-specific interpretations of existing policies.

The following committees may or may not be present, depending on a health plan's corporate structure. Furthermore, these committees may or may not be formal, and may or may not have authority on the health plan's behalf.

Common Corporate Committees

Most companies have certain corporate committees. These committees focus on nonmedical issues relevant to running a business. Although rarely limited to just these three, the most common of these committees are:

- Executive Committee of the Board—provided with board-level decision making authority for issues that must be addressed before a board can meet
- Audit Committee—charged with direct oversight of issues relating to financial statements and relationships with the outside auditing firm
- Compensation Committee—charged with determining the appropriate levels of compensation and incentives to key executives

Quality Management Committee

Usually required under law and/or for accreditation purposes, the quality management committee is essential for overseeing quality management, standard setting, data review, feedback to providers, follow-up, and approval of sanctions. A peer review committee may be a subcommittee of the quality management committee, or it may be separate.

Credentialing Committee

Health plans generally have a credentialing committee charged with ensuring that the providers have the necessary professional qualifications (i.e., credentials) to participate in the plan. This committee may be a subcommittee of the quality management committee, or it may be separate. In states that have carefully defined "due process" requirements for provider termination, this is the committee most likely to take on the responsibility for compliance with those requirements.

Medical Advisory Committee

The purpose of a medical advisory committee is to review general medical management issues brought to it by the medical director. Such issues may include changes in the contract with providers, in compensation, or in authorization procedures. This committee serves as a sounding board for the medical director. Occasionally, it has decision-making authority, but that is rare. In national companies, a local committee may have input for local medical management issues, but a corporate-level medical policy committee generally resolves medical issues that cross all plans (e.g., medical policies regarding new technology).

Utilization Review/Care Management Committee

The medical director may bring utilization or care management issues to this committee. Often this committee is responsible for policies regarding plan coverage. This committee may also review the utilization patterns of the providers and may impose sanctions on providers who use medical resources inappropriately or unwisely.

Sometimes, in reviewing cases for medical necessity, the utilization review committee helps to resolve disputes between the plan and a provider regarding utilization. In large plans, this function may be placed in the hands of various specialty panels charged with reviewing the utilization of consultants (i.e., specialty physicians). The committee may be part of the medical advisory committee, or it may be freestanding.

Pharmacy and Therapeutics Committee

Plans that offer significant pharmacy benefits to their members often have a pharmacy and therapeutics committee. This committee is usually charged with developing a formulary (a list of drugs approved for prescription by plan physicians), reviewing changes to the formulary, and, in smaller plans, examining abnormal prescription utilization patterns by providers. This committee is usually freestanding. In national MCOs, the formulary is usually not subject to local input.

Medical Grievance Review Committee

For HMOs in most states and for members covered under any federal health plan, including Medicare, health plans must establish a separate committee to review member grievances that pertain to medical management or coverage determinations. A particular grievance must be investigated mostly by health care professionals whose specialty encompasses the medical condition at issue. Therefore, most health care professional members will attend a committee meeting only if their specialty is appropriate to the grievance under review. The health care professionals investigating the grievance should not have participated in the member's medical care; if the grievance is significant, it may be necessary to have practitioners who are not associated with the plan look at the validity of the grievance.

Related to the grievance review process is the process for external review of appeals. In states that do not require external reviews, the reviews may be performed by a contracted group of independent physicians. In states that do, the states themselves usually define the independent review organization and require that it not be part of the plan's committee structure. Under ERISA, even self-funded health benefits plans are subject to requirements for reviews of denied coverage for medical services.

Corporate Compliance Committee

Corporate compliance activities are directed toward ensuring conformance to legal and regulatory requirements and preventing and detecting illegal behavior. Corporate compliance programs usually include a special compliance committee that is responsible for creating standards of conduct for employees and also creating policies and procedures specifically designed to ensure compliance with pertinent regulations, such as Medicare Advantage and HIPAA requirements.

CONCLUSION

An understanding of the common types of MCOs and IDSs, as well as their basic management, is required to understand any of the components of managed care. The continuing evolution of managed care results in ever-expanding and mutating definitions and operational structures. Although traditional terms such as "health maintenance organization" and "preferred provider organization" retain considerable utility, the terminology in this industry has an underlying instability. This characteristic should be looked on not as a hindrance toward understanding but as a mark of the exciting and dynamic nature of the industry.

This chapter is adapted in part from E. R. Wagner and P.R. Kongstvedt, "Types of Managed Health Care Plans and Integrated Healthcare Delivery Systems," in *The Essentials of Managed Health Care,* 5th edition, ed. P. R. Kongstvedt (Sudbury, MA: Jones & Bartlett Publishers, 2007).

Network Management and Reimbursement

Managed care organizations (MCOs) such as health maintenance organizations (HMOs) or preferred provider organizations (PPOs) provide for the financing and delivery of health care services through networks of providers under contract. Service plans as described in Chapter 2 also have contracted networks even if they have few other managed care features. Most non-HMO types of MCOs, such as point-of-service (POS) plans and various types of service or indemnity insurance health plans, also provide financial coverage of some type for health care rendered by providers who are not under contract, though almost always with limits on how much will be paid for any service. Integrated delivery systems (IDSs) provide health care services under managed care, although they do not necessarily provide for the financing of those services.

The contracted provider networks are referred to collectively as the health care delivery system or simply as "the network." The network is composed principally of physicians, nonphysician professionals (e.g., psychologists), hospitals, providers of various ancillary services such as diagnostic services (e.g., radiology and laboratory services) and therapeutic services (e.g., physical therapy), and pharmacies, among others (Figure 3–1).

GENERAL CONTRACTING ISSUES

It is the presence of a contract at all that defines an MCO—if there are no contracts between the plan and a network of providers, then it is not an MCO, but rather some type of indemnity insurance plan (Figure 3–2).

Definitions

The contract must specify what it covers and what it does not cover. Items that require definition include the following:

- Plan components such as member, subscriber, medical director, provider, payer, physician, and hospital
- Routine medical services and experimental and/or investigational services
- "Medically necessary" and "emergent or urgent" medical services
- Services that providers are expected to provide under the contract
- Services that providers are not expected to provide under the contract

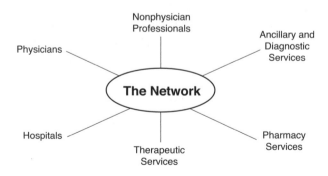

FIGURE 3–1 Components of a Provider Network

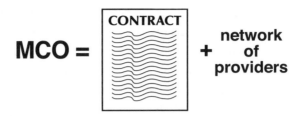

FIGURE 3–2 The New Math

Standard MCO Contract Provisions

Required Qualifications and Credentials

The contract must make it absolutely clear that the provider must have, and maintain, certain qualifications and credentials to remain under contract to the MCO. Common examples for physicians include an unrestricted license to practice medicine, hospital privileges (i.e., the right to admit patients), malpractice insurance, and board certification. Common examples for hospitals include certification by appropriate accreditation agencies, full participation in Medicare (and often Medicaid), and maintenance of licensure.

Required Compliance with the MCO's Utilization and Quality Management Programs

The contract describes the management programs of the MCO that focus on resource utilization and quality of care. In addition, it describes the obligations of both the provider and the MCO under these programs.

"Hold Harmless" and "No Balance Billing" Clauses

A highly important section of the contract outlines the provider's agreement to accept as payment in full for medical services provided to MCO members the amount that the MCO determines to be appropriate. For example, if a physician normally charges $100 for an office visit but the MCO's fee schedule allows only $75, then the physician agrees that under no circumstances will he or she bill the member for the $25 difference; in other words, the provider will "hold the member harmless" from any additional payment. The provider agrees to accept payment only from the MCO, except for the portion that is the clear obligation of the member, such as a copayment (e.g., a $20-per-visit payment), coinsurance (e.g., 20 percent of the total allowed by the MCO, *not* the total originally billed by the provider), or a specified deductible (e.g., a $500 amount that the member must pay for health care services before any insurance coverage begins to apply). The provision applies to hospitals in the same way.

This clause also prohibits the provider from billing the member even in the event that the MCO does not pay the fee at all (if, for example, the MCO refused to pay because the service was not authorized for coverage). All state and federal regulatory agencies require the "no balance billing" clause for contracts between providers and the MCO for almost all forms of MCOs. It is an absolute requirement in HMOs and a likely requirement for most PPOs and service plans as well (see Chapter 2). This clause will also apply in the case of an MCO filing bankruptcy or going out of business, though enforcement is often very difficult in those rare situations.

Payment or Reimbursement Terms

The actual financial terms of a provider's contract with an MCO change periodically. Because it is far easier to change an appendix or attachment than to amend an entire contract, the reimbursement terms usually appear in an appendix or attachment to the contract.

Other-Party Liability: Subrogation and Coordination of Benefits

In some cases, there may be more than one payer responsible for coverage of medical services. For example, a man may have health insurance through work, whereas his wife also has health insurance through her own place of employment. If the couple's child receives medical care, which parent's insurance will be primarily responsible and which parent's insurance will be secondarily responsible (Figure 3–3)? Further, can both policies be used to increase the total amount of insurance coverage available? Similarly, which insurance will cover medical services provided to an MCO member if those services are the result of an accident (e.g., an automobile accident in which the auto insurance pays for part of the medical services)? The contract sets out the basic rules for dealing with such situations.

Term and Termination

One section of the contract specifies how long the contract is for and under what circumstances either party may terminate it. Termination provisions have become

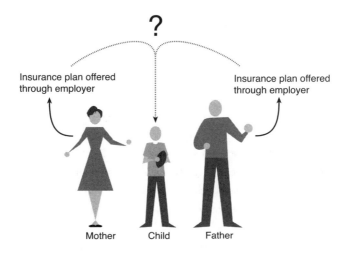

FIGURE 3–3 The Question Raised by Dual Insurance Coverage

very complex in many states. In past decades, either party could terminate the contract simply by giving adequate notice (i.e., notifying the other party as far ahead of time as the contract requires for such notification, such as 90 days). Some states require MCOs that no longer want a provider's services to furnish the provider with the reasons for termination, and a few states have created due process requirements that allow a terminated provider to dispute the termination. No laws have been enacted that require providers to furnish reasons for wishing to terminate a contract with an MCO or that allow the MCO to dispute the termination.

There are three common categories of reasons for termination:

1. *Inadequate quality of care.* An MCO must take action to remove an incompetent provider from the network. Such terminations are reportable to the appropriate government agencies (e.g., the state department of licensure or health; the National Practitioner Data Bank).

2. *Failure to meet recredentialing requirements.* Providers may have a change in their professional status. For example, a physician may fail to requalify for board certification (requalification is required every 10 years in most specialties) or may have had his or her license restricted.

3. *Business reasons.* An MCO or a provider may conclude that having no contract is preferable to the terms of the existing contract. In the case of an MCO, the MCO's medical managers may have determined that a particular provider's practice behavior is unsuitable for a managed care environment. It

is this third category that has created great distress among providers and has led several states to pass laws that inhibit MCOs from terminating physicians for business reasons.

PHYSICIANS

In general, physicians are health care professionals who have a license to prescribe medications, privileges to admit patients to hospitals, and other related attributes. They most commonly have earned the degree of medical doctor (MD) or doctor of osteopathy (DO). In many states, and often by convention, other professionals, such as a doctor of chiropractic (DC), may also carry the designation of physician. This follows common usage in the managed care industry.

There are many ways to classify physicians. It is most common to differentiate physicians based on whether they are functioning in the role of primary care physician (PCP) or specialty care physician. There is a third distinction that is really a variation of specialty care physician. This is a form of a specialty care physician organization that is highly focused on providing a particular type of health care. The distinctions between these types of physicians are not always clear. They remain useful, however, because many aspects of managed care are based on them.

Primary Care Physicians

In virtually all health care systems, care rendered by physicians in the specialties of family practice, internal medicine, and pediatrics is considered primary care. General practitioners (i.e., physicians who have not obtained full residency training beyond their internships) may also be considered PCPs, but few MCOs contract with them except in rural or underserved areas where there may not be a sufficient number of residency-trained PCPs to provide care to all MCO members.

Many OB/GYN specialists feel that they too deliver primary care to their patients because a young woman's gynecologist is often the only physician she sees for many years. This may be true in the case of generally healthy young women, but it is not always so for those who have medical problems that do not involve medical care unique to women. Currently, virtually all MCOs allow female members to have direct access to OB/GYNs. It should be noted that, in addition to simple market demands, many states have passed laws requiring MCOs to allow direct access to OB/GYNs. For clinical care that is beyond the scope of normal OB/GYN practice, the member will usually see a PCP for treatment or referral to another specialist.

Role of the Primary Care Physician

In all types of MCOs and IDSs, the PCP's role is extremely important. Many HMOs require enrollees to visit their PCP to obtain either direct care or a referral authorization for specialty care. Called a gatekeeper or coordinating physician, this PCP coordinates all services for the enrollees in his or her practice. Even when there is no such requirement, many U.S. citizens receive most of their regular health care from PCPs.

Although it is common for PCPs to be trained in primary care, there are certain clinical circumstances under which it is better for a specialist to act as the PCP. For example (as discussed in Chapter 4), a patient with severe heart disease is usually better managed by a cardiologist for all medical problems than by a general internist, because almost any clinical condition will have an impact on the heart in such a patient. Specialty-trained internists frequently function as PCPs as well. Some confusion may arise, however, if the same physician is functioning as a PCP for some members and a specialty care physician for others.

Nonphysician or Midlevel Practitioners in Primary Care

Among the nonphysician or midlevel practitioners in primary care are physician's assistants and nurse practitioners. There are several different types of nurse practitioner designations, each having a different focus and training; for example, there are advanced practice nurses, nurse-midwives, nurse-anesthetists, and clinical nurse specialists. The rise of retail or convenience clinics, clinics located in drug or grocery stores that deliver routine care (e.g., for immunizations or for a sore throat), are almost always staffed by nurse practitioners rather than physicians. MCOs have been quick to contract with these clinics to provide routine care at lower costs than typical physician or urgent care centers.

Nonphysician providers may play an especially important role in the management of chronically ill patients. They may coordinate care or function as case managers for patients with diseases such as chronic asthma, diabetes, and the like. In a similar vein, nonphysician providers may take a key role in managing the care of high-risk patients, using practice protocols for disease prevention and health maintenance in this population. Certified nurse-midwives may provide not only services for routine deliveries but also primary gynecological care using practice guidelines and protocols.

The presence of such nonphysician practitioners is generally an asset in managed care because they are able to deliver excellent primary care and provide more health maintenance and health promotion services, and they tend to spend more time with patients.

Specialty Care Physicians

Also commonly referred to as specialists, specialty care physicians (e.g., cardiologists, surgeons) provide specialty health care services, even if some of those services are essentially the same as those delivered by PCPs. In HMOs at least, a physician who is not a PCP will be considered a specialty care physician. Other types of MCOs may or may not differentiate between specialty and primary care. As noted earlier, in an HMO, it is possible for a single physician to be both, although rarely for the same patient. For example, a cardiologist may be the PCP for an enrolled panel of members but also serve as a specialty care physician to other PCPs. This cardiologist cannot see a member as a PCP, however, and then refer the same member back to himself or herself as a specialty care physician (thus generating two bills). Even in HMOs, and commonly in other types of MCOs, it is becoming increasingly common for specialty care physicians to function as PCPs for those members with significant chronic illnesses, even if they do not otherwise function as PCPs.

"Carve-Out" and Specialty Care Services

Not only specialty care physicians practicing individually or in medical groups but also specialty care organizations may provide specialty services. In these cases, the specialty care services focus on defined disease states or medical conditions. The specialty care organization may be a company, a large medical group, or a specialty independent practice association (IPA). For example, it is common for MCOs to contract with a company to provide all behavioral health and substance abuse services. Less commonly, an MCO may contract with an organization for all services related to renal dialysis or cancer care. This is often referred to as a "carve-out" service, in that the costs and mechanisms for managing the service have been carved out of the overall budget and medical management program and are handled separately.

Hospital-Based Physicians

A unique type of specialist is the hospital-based physician (HBP). Broadly speaking, HBPs fall into one of four specialties:

- Radiology
- Anesthesiology
- Pathology
- Hospitalist

All acute care medical/surgical hospitals have the first three specialties, and many large hospitals have the fourth as well. There are two defining features of an HBP. The first is that there is usually no competition within a hospital for the particular specialty of the HBP. For example, one single radiology group may provide all professional services for inpatient and outpatient radiology at the hospital. Even in the rare instances in which there is more than one group or different private practitioners providing services (more common for anesthesia than for the other three specialties), there is some system in place to determine how services will be divided up, and in no case does the patient have any choice. The second defining feature is that it is essentially not possible to receive inpatient care without incurring charges from one or more of the first three types of HBP.

Outpatient radiology and elective ambulatory procedures that require anesthesia may be done on a more selective basis, however. Pathology fees associated with elective outpatient laboratory and pathology may likewise be more selective by requiring only the use of contracted providers.

Hospitalists are different from the other three types of HBPs. Hospitalists are physicians who concentrate solely on the day-to-day management of inpatient care, excluding certain focused types of cases such as childbirth or transplantation. In large hospitals with very active intensive care units, a specialized type of hospitalist, called an intensivist, focuses only on caring for the critically ill, regardless of whether or not there is also a hospitalist managing non-intensive inpatient care.

Contracting with the other types of HBPs regarding hospital-associated care can present challenges to MCOs because they hold what amounts to a monopoly for their particular types of inpatient services. Lack of a contract may even create a barrier to contracting with a hospital that is otherwise willing to agree to contract.

Credentialing

An MCO has an obligation to verify that the physicians in its network meet the professional standards that it has established for its participating providers. The credentialing process actually begins before a physician receives a contract in the first place, and recredentialing takes place every 2 years.

An MCO is generally required to perform what is referred to as "primary source" credentialing, that is, obtaining documents directly from pertinent agencies or schools. But because the process of credentialing often varies little from MCO to MCO, and to reduce the burden on both MCOs and physicians, MCOs frequently rely on a third-party credentialing verification organization, or CVO, to perform primary credentialing on a physician. The CVO must itself be certified by the appropriate certification agency.

The common basic elements of initial credentialing (i.e., the credentialing that occurs before a physician joins the network) include the following:

- Demographic information
  - ➤ Full name
  - ➤ Date and place of birth
  - ➤ Gender
  - ➤ Home and e-mail addresses
- Office information
  - ➤ Location and telephone numbers of all offices
  - ➤ General information such as hours, on-call coverage, limitations, and so forth
  - ➤ Billing and payment information
- Training (copy of certificates)
  - ➤ Location of training
  - ➤ Type of training
- Specialty care board eligibility or certification (copy of certificate)
- Current state medical license (copy of certificate)
  - ➤ Restrictions
  - ➤ History of loss of license in any state
- Medical license numbers in all states where provider is licensed
- National Provider Identifier (NPI) as required under the Health Insurance Portability and Accountability Act (HIPAA). Previously issued Medicare, Medicaid, and other provider identification numbers may also be requested even though they were phased out by the NPI.
- Drug Enforcement Agency (DEA) and state-controlled substance (if required by state) numbers and copies of certificates
- Federal tax identification number
- Social security number
- Hospital privileges
  - ➤ Names of hospitals
  - ➤ Scope of practice privileges
- Work history for past 5–10 years
- Malpractice insurance
  - ➤ Name of insurance carrier
  - ➤ Currency of coverage (copy of face sheet)
  - ➤ Scope of coverage (i.e., financial limits and procedures covered)

- Malpractice history
  - Pending claims
  - Successful claims against the physician, either judged or settled
- Professional references
- Yes/No questions regarding:
  - Limitations or suspensions of privileges
  - Suspension from participation in any government programs
  - Suspension or restriction of DEA license
  - Cancellation of malpractice insurance
  - Felony conviction
  - Drug or alcohol abuse
  - Chronic or debilitating illnesses

Additional elements of initial credentialing that are not always required, but increasingly asked, include:

- Use of midlevel practitioners (e.g., physician's assistants or clinical nurse practitioners)
- In-office surgery capabilities
- In-office testing capabilities
- Languages spoken
- Areas of special medical interest
- Continuing medical education

The MCO obtains the credentialing information from the physician, from a CVO, or directly from the relevant agencies (e.g., the physician's medical school). In addition, the MCO (as well as all hospitals) must query the National Practitioner Data Bank (NPDB). Created under the Health Care Quality Improvement Act of 1986 (HCQIA), with final regulations published in 1989,[1] the NPDB serves as a central repository of information on the following topics:

- Malpractice payments made for the benefit of physicians, dentists, and other health care practitioners
- Licensure actions taken by state medical boards and state boards of dentistry against physicians and dentists, and other health care practitioners who are licensed or otherwise authorized by a state to provide health care services
- Actions taken as a result of professional reviews, primarily against physicians and dentists by hospitals and other health care entities, including HMOs, group practices, and professional societies

- Actions taken by the Drug Enforcement Agency
- Medicare/Medicaid participation exclusions

The enabling act, HCQIA, provides for qualified immunity from antitrust lawsuits for credentialing activities, as well as professional medical staff sanctions, when the terms of the act are followed. Information reported to the NPDB is considered confidential and may not be disclosed except as needed to:

- Hospitals
- Other health care entities with formal peer review
- Professional societies with formal peer review
- Boards of medical/dental examiners and other health care practitioner state licensing boards
- Plaintiffs' attorneys or plaintiffs representing themselves (limited)
- Health care practitioners (self-query)
- Researchers (statistical data only)

Also created under HIPAA is the Healthcare Integrity and Protection Data Bank (HIPDB), created to combat fraud and abuse in health insurance and health care delivery. The HIPDB is a national data collection program for the reporting and disclosure of certain final adverse actions taken against health care providers, suppliers, and practitioners (excluding settlements in which no findings of liability have been made). It is to contain information about:

- Civil judgments against health care providers, suppliers, or practitioners in federal or state courts related to the delivery of health care items or services
- Federal or state criminal convictions against health care providers, suppliers, or practitioners related to the delivery of health care items or services
- Actions by federal or state agencies responsible for the licensing and certification of health care providers, suppliers, or practitioners
- Exclusion of health care providers, suppliers, or practitioners from participation in federal or state health care programs
- Any other adjudicated actions or decisions that the secretary of the Department of Health and Human Services establishes through regulations

Access to information from the HIPDB is limited to:

- Federal and state government agencies
- Health plans
- Health care practitioners/providers/suppliers (self-query)
- Researchers (statistical data only)

After the physician becomes part of the network, recredentialing occurs every 2 years. The credentialing information may be simply updated by the physician directly or through the credentialing verification organization. At the time of recredentialing, many MCOs add information gleaned from quality assurance surveys and member satisfaction surveys. It is also necessary to requery the NPDB and the HIPDB. The basic elements of recredentialing include the following:

- Current status of state medical license (copy of current valid certificate)
  1. Restrictions
  2. History of loss or restriction of license in any state
- Copy of current valid DEA certificate
- Any changes to their NPI, or any additional NPIs the provider my have been issued
- Status of hospital privileges
  1. Names of hospitals
  2. Scope of practice privileges
- Current malpractice insurance status
  1. Name of insurance carrier
  2. Currency of coverage (copy of face sheet)
  3. Scope of coverage (financial limits and procedures covered)
- Malpractice history over past 2 years
  1. Pending claims
  2. Successful claims against the physician, either judged or settled
- Yes/No questions regarding:
  1. Limitations or suspensions of privileges
  2. Suspension from government programs
  3. Suspension or restriction of DEA license
  4. Cancellation of malpractice insurance
  5. Felony conviction
  6. Drug or alcohol abuse
  7. Chronic or debilitating illnesses

The National Provider Identifier

As noted in the list of information gathered in the credentialing process, HIPAA called for the use of the NPI beginning in 2007 (2008 for small health plans). The NPI replaced all other forms of provider identifiers, such as the Medicare universal provider identification numbers (UPIN), Blue Cross and Blue Shield numbers, health plan provider numbers, Medicaid numbers, and so forth. The only provider numbers that were not affected were the taxpayer identifying number and the DEA number for providers who prescribe or administer prescription drugs. The NPI is a 10-digit number that is unique and never-ending in that once assigned a NPI, the provider will use that identifier for all transactions regardless of location, plan type, or anything else.

Electronic Connectivity

Although still not common, as pressures to lower administrative costs continue and as the need for more accurate and efficient business transactions becomes acute, some MCOs are considering requiring electronic communication of basic transactions (e.g., claims billing and authorizations) as a condition of contract renewal. This is not dissimilar to the requirements that Medicare currently has for participating providers to submit claims electronically (requirements that are largely met via the use of third-party billing services). In addition, and again with Medicare leading the way, a requirement to use electronic prescribing is being considered by some health plans. In all cases, because of HIPAA, there are uniform electronic standards for these types of electronic transactions.

Electronic Medical Records

The use of electronic medical records (EMRs) in physician's offices remains low except in relatively large medical groups. Hindered both by a lack of mandated electronic standards and by the cost to install it, plus the time investment required to learn to use it, smaller medical groups and solo practitioners have resisted its use. Although the federal government has as yet declined to mandate standards, it has established an office that officially sanctions standards, so there is at least an informally "blessed" standard for each element. MCOs often include a financial incentive for the use of EMRs, usually through a performance bonus, as discussed later in this chapter.

Reimbursement of Physicians

HMOs frequently pay their physicians, especially PCPs, according to some form of risk-based reimbursement system (i.e., reimbursement has some element of risk for medical expenses). Less commonly, specialty care physicians may receive payment for their services under some form of risk-based reimbursement. Other types of MCOs rarely use risk-based reimbursement and in fact are usually prohibited from doing so by law (i.e., most states only allow HMOs to place providers at any risk for medical costs). A different type of performance-based compensation for both physicians and hospitals is referred to as pay-for-performance (P4P) and is discussed later in this chapter. P4P may be used by any type of MCO.

The compensation of physicians working under direct contract to MCOs rather than providing services through an intermediary differs from the compensation of individual physicians in organized groups, staff models, or IDSs. It is possible and even common to use these methods of reimbursement for an individual physician in such groups. For example, a medical group might blend the three basic forms of compensation—capitation, fee-for-service (FFS), and salary—to pay individual physicians no matter how the group itself receives payment.

The objective of most managed care reimbursement systems is to better align the compensation of physicians with the overall goals of managed care. By itself, it is unlikely that any compensation system will have much of an impact, however. A reimbursement system is simply one of the many tools available in managed care and usually does not achieve the desired goals in the absence of other vital tools, such as competent management of utilization and quality. Although there are few basic ways of reimbursing physicians and other professionals, there are countless variations on themes and numerous combinations. In addition, withholds or risk and incentive compensation may be applied to any method or combination of methods in HMOs.

Managed care is marked by a high degree of change and variation. Change is produced by market forces, new managed care practices, new laws and regulations (especially in Medicare and Medicaid), and uncountable other factors. As a result, provider types and the reimbursement mechanisms are rarely found in their pure form.

Capitation

Although FFS remains the most common form of physician reimbursement, capitation is a powerful and popular option for HMOs. It involves fixed payments made on a per-member per-month (PMPM) basis regardless of the use of services. In other words, the physician receives a fixed amount of money each month for every member of the HMO who enrolls in that physician's panel of patients. Whether the member seeks care every day or never seeks care at all, the amount of money that the physician receives does not vary.

The actual capitation fees are usually adjusted based on the age and sex of each enrolled member, because there is some correlation between those factors and utilization (i.e., medical costs). In general, older members use more health care services than younger members, and young women use more services than young men. Capitation fees, in rare cases, are adjusted based on other factors, such as geographic location. For technical reasons, it is difficult to adjust capitation based on how sick a patient is, but there is some experimentation with it, and adjustments based on level of sickness may become more common in the future.

The key to making capitation work is to receive fees from a large number of members, most of whom will not need extensive (and expensive) services. Because the members of a "gatekeeper" type of HMO must select a single PCP to provide and coordinate care, ensuring that they are counted only once, capitation is most easily applied to PCPs in such health plans. Capitation may be used for physicians in high-volume specialties as well, but for specialists, there must be some mechanism to ensure that, except in special circumstances, the members for whom the HMO is making capitation payments will not seek or receive services from non-capitated providers.

Capitation payments made directly to providers may be subject to a withhold. For example, the HMO may hold back 10 percent of the total amount of capitation to be paid to a provider to cover unexpectedly high rates of utilization. Withholds are less common than they once were because many HMOs now prefer to base their programs primarily on incentives rather than penalties.

Incentive payments are common in HMOs, at least for PCPs. In general, the incentive payment is a reward for providers who keep down utilization or medical costs. In a typical arrangement, a pool of money is set aside in an amount determined by the number of members. The HMO applies the money during the year against expenses in a defined category, such as referral or hospital costs, and then distributes the remainder at the end of the year (in part or in whole) to the physicians based on utilization patterns either of the entire panel of physicians or of each individual physician. Incentive programs for physicians that are based on high-quality care, accessibility, and member satisfaction, known as pay-for-performance (P4P) programs, are becoming more common. Because P4P programs can be applied to physicians and hospitals in any type of MCO, they are discussed later in the chapter.

The variations on the theme of capitation are numerous (Figure 3–4). For example, although rarely used, contact capitation can be used to reimburse specialty care physicians. In this system, patients choose specialists of the kind they need to see, and the HMO then pays each specialist a percentage of the total capitation

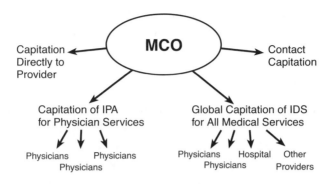

FIGURE 3–4 Examples of Types of Capitation

dollars that the HMO had set aside to cover the care that its members might need from such a specialist. For example, if 100 members received orthopedic care from six orthopedists, then the HMO would distribute the total capitation dollars to those orthopedists based on the percentage of the 100 members whom each orthopedist saw (e.g., if one saw 15 members, that orthopedist would receive 15 percent of the total amount available for orthopedic care). Adjustments are also made for severity of illness, duration of the episode of care, and other variables, increasing the complexity of the system. Contact capitation requires very large membership bases and highly sophisticated computer systems.

Global capitation differs from ordinary capitation in that the provider receiving the capitation payment under global capitation may not be the provider actually delivering the health care services. In a global capitation system, the HMO covers all or most medical costs through capitation payments to a large, organized medical group or an IDS—rarely, if ever, to individual physicians or small medical groups. The large group receives capitation payments that cover all the services it provides, as well as any costs from services provided from outside the group. In other words, the globally capitated medical group is responsible for all the medical costs of the HMO members. This form of reimbursement is manageable only by very large groups or IDSs, and even then, its track record has been very poor; many such groups have failed because of their inability to manage the risk for medical costs.

It is common for an IPA to receive global capitation payments on behalf of all the physicians in the IPA, even if the IPA does not in turn make global capitation payments to the individual providers or medical groups. In fact, it is the business of most IPAs to accept capitation payments for the entire network and then apply the more common forms of reimbursement (i.e., individual capitation or FFS) to compensate individual physicians within the IPA. In the same way, certain group model HMOs use global capitation to reimburse the medical group for medical costs, even though the medical group itself pays individual physicians via salary.

Fee-for-Service

While remaining a significant form of reimbursement in HMOs, fee-for-service (FFS) is nearly the only form of reimbursement in PPOs, service plans, and indemnity plans. Even HMOs that use a capitation system for PCPs usually reimburse referral specialists on a FFS basis. In POS plans, it is difficult, if not impossible, to predict actual in-network utilization for each member, making capitation an unsuitable form of compensation for providers. Consequently, many of these plans reimburse even PCPs on a FFS basis. Although somewhat less conducive to managed care than is capitation, FFS is not necessarily unsuitable for managed care.

If not managed properly, a FFS system can lead to higher costs than would occur under capitation. Therefore, it is common for HMOs that use a FFS system to place the fees at some form of risk for the provider. A withhold on a percentage of the fees is the most common mechanism, as discussed in the section on capitation. If utilization exceeds that anticipated in the budget, the MCO uses the withhold to cover the cost overage; if utilization is below that anticipated, the withhold is paid out to providers (or at least those providers who have lower than budgeted medical costs). Some MCOs reduce fees if utilization becomes excessive. Other MCOs have experimented with global fees (i.e., a single fee for a visit or procedure regardless of how much or how little care the patient receives during that visit); this approach has had some success in preventing cost increases resulting from the use of fee codes that pay more.

The methods used to determine what fees to pay for each procedure or visit vary from MCO to MCO. In the past, MCOs often determined fees based on the "usual, customary, or reasonable" fees for services in that area, but over the past two decades, this method became synonymous with uncontrolled fee inflation. Therefore, all MCOs now use some form of fee schedule, setting a maximum amount that a physician will be paid for each individual procedure or service. Physicians under contract to an MCO agree to accept the established amount as payment in full (except for any copayment or coinsurance that the member must pay) and not charge the member the difference between the established amount and what the physicians normally ask.

The use of a relative value scale (RVS) to determine fees is quite common. The MCO assigns a value to each procedure or visit code and determines the fee by multiplying a set dollar amount against the relative value. For example, a procedure may have a relative value of 4.5, and the fee is calculated by multiplying $10 by 4.5, resulting in a fee of $45. (These numbers are for illustration purposes only and do not represent actual relative values or monetary multipliers.)

The most common type of RVS is the resource-based relative value scale (RBRVS) developed by the predecessor of the Centers for Medicare & Medicaid Services (CMS) for use in the Medicare program. Before the development of the RBRVS, most fee schedules and even routine RVSs were based on historical charge patterns, in which the fees for surgical and procedural services were higher than the fees for so-called cognitive (i.e., "thinking") services. For example, 20 minutes of surgery might generate a fee of $800, whereas 20 minutes of time with an internist in the office might generate a fee of $45. The RBRVS was created to address this imbalance by lowering the relative values of many procedural services and raising the relative values of many cognitive services. Although procedures still generate substantially higher fees than do cognitive services, some of the disparity has been reduced. Many MCOs simply adopt the RBRVS as CMS issues and updates, and then use it to calculate provider fees (though the monetary multipliers used differ among the MCOs).

Finally, as cost sharing has been steadily increasing, providers of all types have found it increasingly important to collect the patient's portion of the fee at the time of service. This is particularly the case in consumer-directed health plans (CDHPs) or high-deductible health plans (HDHPs). In the case of both CDHPs and HDHPs, the patient has a substantial deductible, often up to $1,000, and as all office managers know, the longer an outstanding bill does not get paid, the less likely it becomes that it will ever be paid. Therefore, MCOs have been working on technology that allows a physician's office, through the use of the Internet or a swipe card reader combined with a standard credit card issued by the MCO, to know immediately how much the patient is expected to pay out-of-pocket for any particular visit or procedure. Though still not mainstream, such technology is being increasingly used in FFS payment systems.

Salary

Payment of a salary is the predominant method of physician reimbursement in closed-panel plans and in some group practices or situations in which physicians are employees (e.g., full-time faculty, government-employed physicians, or some full-time hospital-based physicians). The employer may apply withholds to the physician's base salary, and incentive plans are common. In a withhold program, the employer holds back a small percentage of the salary (e.g., 10 percent). If medical costs exceed those anticipated, the employer uses the withheld amount to help cover the increased costs. If medical costs are as expected or below, the physician receives the withheld amount.

An incentive program is similar but may encompass more than measurements of medical costs. For example, an MCO or IDS may have a program in which it is possible for employed physicians to receive a bonus of as much as 10–20 percent of their base salary if they keep medical costs within anticipated limits, make every effort to ensure patient satisfaction, are very productive, comply with quality management programs, and fulfill other requirements established by the MCO or IDS. Incentive programs are more common than withhold programs, though in fact the difference may be more a question of wording than of functioning.

Stop-Loss Protection

It is in the interest of both the MCO and the physicians to prevent one or two very costly cases from inflicting a financial penalty on an individual physician. Therefore, in most cases of risk-based reimbursement, there is a limit on a physician's exposure to financial risk. Reaching that limit activates the physician's stop-loss protection. Such protection may be as simple as limiting any financial risk to the amount of the withhold, if one exists. In other cases, such as where global capitation is involved, the degree of risk can be significantly higher (involving large sums of money) and may require the purchase of special insurance, sometimes referred to as stop-loss insurance or reinsurance.

In general, "stop-loss" means that at some point, the amount of costs generated is no longer used to measure the performance or determine the reimbursement of a physician. Specific stop-loss protection shields the physician from high medical costs resulting from an individual patient's case, whereas aggregate stop-loss protection shields the physician from a high total cost for the physician's entire panel of patients. The aim of both types of stop-loss protection is the same: to prevent high costs associated with untypical cases from having an adverse effect on the physician's reimbursement.

Legislation and Regulation Applicable to Physician Incentive Programs

Beginning in the 1990s, the federal government and many (but not all) state governments passed laws and created regulations that affect physician incentive programs. These apply primarily to capitation programs and to incentive programs that increase the income of a physician who provides fewer services. (Of course, there are no such regulations placed upon FFS systems because they reward physicians for doing more, not less, and the provision of more care is supposedly less likely to harm patients.) State laws and regulations that are in force show little consistency from one state to another, but in general, they focus on the disclosure of financial incentives.

CMS has implemented regulations that place limits on physician incentive programs in Medicare and Medicaid MCOs on a national basis. In general, these regulations outline a set of conditions that may be considered to place a physician at "significant financial risk," conditions that vary based on several factors (e.g., the size of the medical group at risk for medical costs, the percentage of total compensation at risk for medical costs). If there is a significant financial risk, then the MCO must provide specific levels and types of stop-loss insurance and may need to undertake special types of consumer satisfaction surveys. In addition, the federal regulations require disclosure of each physician's amount and type of financial risk, at least in the case of physicians providing care for Medicare and/or Medicaid patients.

HOSPITALS AND INSTITUTIONS

Obviously, an MCO needs to have hospitals and institutional providers in its service area (e.g., acute care hospitals, skilled and intermediate care facilities, and all types of ambulatory facilities). Every MCO must ensure that all its members have access to reasonably convenient acute care, especially emergency care. The licensure bodies for MCOs, often state departments of insurance, usually have requirements for the maximum permissible amount of time or distance that a member must travel to receive care; for example, it is common to require a drive time of 30 minutes or less to access an acute care hospital and emergency department. If an MCO is unable to provide access to a contracted facility within those time or distance limits, the state may refuse to license the MCO or at least not allow the MCO to market services in any geographic area in which access to services is inadequate. Employers or purchasers may have similar or even stricter requirements for access.

Access is also a function of the services provided. For example, two nearby hospitals may differ in the services they offer; only one of the two may offer obstetric services, whereas the other might be the sole provider of trauma services. An MCO must take the types of services into account, as well as location, when building its network of providers.

The types of institutional providers that MCO members must have access to include subacute care facilities, rehabilitation centers, skilled and intermediate care facilities, and ambulatory surgery (or more accurately, ambulatory procedure) facilities. Skilled and intermediate care facilities, often referred to as "nursing homes," play an important role in the Medicare and Medicaid programs and also have a place in commercial programs. Ambulatory surgical centers, or outpatient surgery centers, may be part of a hospital, may be owned by a hospital, or may be freestanding. Location is less important for these facilities because virtually all care is elective, and therefore, access to them is not urgent. Specific coverage for non-acute care varies from plan to plan.

Reimbursement Methods

A number of reimbursement methods are available to MCOs in contracting with hospitals and other health care institutions (except in those few states where regulations diminish or prohibit creativity), and it is common to find an MCO using more than one method to reimburse a single institution. Exhibit 3–1 describes the various types of reimbursement methods.

Straight Charges

The simplest payment method in health care is to pay straight charges (i.e., charges undiscounted in any way). It is also obviously the most expensive. An

EXHIBIT 3–1

Reimbursement Methods

Straight Charges
Discount on Charges
    Straight discount on charges
    Sliding scale discount on charges
Per Diem Charges
    Straight per diem charges
    Sliding scale per diem
    Differential by day in hospital
Diagnosis-Related Groups (DRGs)
Medicare Severity Diagnosis-Related Groups (MS-DRGs)
Case Rates and Package Pricing
Capitation or Percentage of Revenue
Contact Capitation
Periodic Interim Payments and Cash Advances
Package Pricing or Bundled Charges

MCO will agree to pay straight charges only in the event that it is unable to obtain any form of discount but wants to have a contract with a "no balance billing" clause in it to meet reserve and licensure requirements.

Discount on Charges

Straight discount on charges. Another possible method is to discount charges by a straight percentage. In this method, the hospital submits its bill in the full amount, and the MCO discounts it by the previously agreed percentage and then pays it. The hospital accepts this payment as payment in full. The amount of discount that can be obtained will depend on the factors discussed earlier, such as the degree of competitiveness in the market, the desire of the hospital to receive patients from the MCO, and so forth. The straight discount method is common in markets with low levels of managed care penetration but is uncommon in markets with high levels of managed care penetration.

Sliding scale discount on charges. In markets with few MCOs but some level of competitiveness between hospitals, sliding scale discounts are an option. With a sliding scale, the percentage discount reflects the total volume of services provided. For example, there may be a 20 percent reduction in charges for 0–200 total bed days per year, with incremental increases in the discount as the number of bed days increases—up to a maximum percentage. An interim percentage discount is usually negotiated, and the parties reconcile at the end of the year based on the final total volume.

Whether to lump admissions and outpatient procedures together or deal with them separately is not as important as making sure that the parties deal with them both. With the continually climbing cost of outpatient care, an unanticipated overrun in outpatient charges could erase savings obtained from a reduction of inpatient utilization.

Per Diem Charges

Straight per diem charges. A common type of arrangement is for MCOs to reimburse hospitals on the basis of straight per diem (which means "per day") charges. The MCO negotiates a single per diem rate of payment per day in the hospital and pays that rate regardless of any actual charges or costs incurred. The per diem is simply an estimate of the charges or costs for an average day in that hospital minus the level of discount. The key to making a per diem work is predictability. If the MCO and hospital can accurately predict the number and mix of cases, then they can calculate an adequate per diem.

Hospital administrators are often reluctant to include days in the intensive care or obstetric units as part of the base per diem unless there is sufficient volume of regular medical-surgical cases to make the ultimate cost predictable. For a small MCO or one that is not limiting the number of participating hospitals, administrators may be concerned that the MCO will use its hospital for expensive cases at a low per diem while using competing hospitals for less costly cases. In this situation, a good option is to negotiate multiple sets of per diem charges based on service type (e.g., medical-surgical procedures, obstetrics, intensive care, neonatal intensive care, and rehabilitation) or a combination of per diems and a flat case rate for obstetrics (costs are predictable for routine obstetric care, and a flat case rate rewards efficient hospitals).

Some MCOs may also negotiate an agreement by which they reimburse the hospital for certain expensive surgical implants provided at the hospital's actual cost of the implant. Such reimbursement would be limited to a defined list of implants (e.g., inner ear implants) for which the cost to the hospital for the implant is far greater than is recoverable under the per diem arrangement.

Sliding scale per diem.   Like the sliding scale discount on charges, the sliding scale per diem is based on total volume. In this case, the MCO agrees to pay an interim per diem for each day that one of its members spends in the hospital during the year. The more days that the MCO members spend in the hospital during the year, however, the lower the per diem rate. Depending on the total number of bed days or admissions in the year, the MCO will either pay a lump sum settlement at the end of the year or withhold an amount from the final payment to adjust for the actual number of bed days or admissions. It is wise to review and possibly adjust the interim per diem on a quarterly or semiannual basis so as to reduce disparities caused by unexpected changes in utilization patterns.

Differential by day in hospital.   Most hospitalizations are more expensive on the first day. For example, the first day charges for surgical cases include operating suite costs, the operating surgical team costs (nurses and recovery), and so forth. The reimbursement method for such services is generally a variation of the per diem approach, with the first day paid at a higher rate.

Diagnosis-Related Groups and Medicare Severity Diagnosis-Related Groups

MCOs often use diagnosis-related groups (DRGs) for the purpose of reimbursing hospitals. There are publications that contain information on DRG categories, criteria, outliers (cases that may fall into a DRG category but are far more severe and require far longer lengths of stay than the DRG covers), and trim points (the cost or length of stay that triggers supplementation or replacement of the DRG payment by another payment mechanism; applied to outliers) to enable MCOs to negotiate DRG payment rates. A few MCOs base their payments on Medicare rates (or in rare cases, state-regulated rates), but as Medicare payments have dropped below the costs to deliver services, most commercial MCOs pay higher DRG rates than Medicare.

Beginning in 2008 and scheduled for completion in 2009, Medicare will replace standard DRGs with Medicare Severity DRGs (MS-DRGs). MS-DRGs collapse some existing DRGs into fewer categories, while adding DRG codes to account for patients with existing complications or comorbidities (i.e., have multiple chronic medical conditions), or major complications and comorbidities (i.e., have complications from one or more of their multiple chronic medical conditions). This will better align payment to the actual costs to care for such complicated patients. As MS-DRGs are instituted by Medicare, there will be less need for trim points and outlier coverage by Medicare. Commercial MCOs are likely to quickly follow suit. Either way, DRGs are the preferred method of reimbursing hospitals for many MCOs because DRGs place most of the financial risk on the hospital, thereby requiring less medical management by the MCO.

Case Rates and Package Pricing

Whatever mechanism an MCO uses for hospital reimbursement, it may still be necessary to address certain categories of procedures or services and negotiate special rates for those categories. In the area of obstetrics, for example, it is common for an MCO either to negotiate a case rate for a normal vaginal delivery and a case rate for a cesarean section or to negotiate a blended rate for both. In the case of blended case rates (which are much preferred over separate rates for the two types of deliveries because they eliminate any financial incentive to do cesarean sections), the expected reimbursement for each type of delivery is multiplied by the expected (or desired) percentage of utilization. For example, a case rate for vaginal delivery is $3,500, and for cesarean section it is $5,000. Utilization is expected to be 80% vaginal and 20% cesarean section, and therefore the case rate is $3,800 ($3,500 × 0.8 = $2,800; $5,000 × 0.2 = $1,000; $2,800 + $1,000 = $3,800); these numbers are purely hypothetical and do not represent actual costs or payments.

Other common areas in which case rates make sense are procedures at tertiary (i.e., specialty) hospitals; for example, MCOs may establish case rates for coronary artery bypass surgery, heart transplants, obesity surgery, or certain types of cancer treatment. These procedures, although relatively infrequent, are tremendously costly.

Package pricing or bundled case rates are all-inclusive rates paid for both institutional and professional services. The MCO negotiates a flat rate for a procedure (e.g., coronary artery bypass surgery), and that rate covers the fees of all parties who provide services connected with that procedure, including preadmission and postdischarge care. Bundled case rates are not uncommon in teaching facilities, where the faculty members practice as part of the hospital staff and are used to sharing income with the teaching hospital.

Capitation or Percentage of Revenue

As it does with physicians, capitation by an HMO may be used for reimbursement of a hospital or institution on a PMPM basis to cover all the facility's costs in providing medical care for a defined population of members. The payment may be varied according to the age and sex of patients but does not fluctuate with premium revenue. A percentage of revenue plan, on the other hand, involves paying a fixed percentage of premium revenue (i.e., a percentage of the collected premium payments) to the hospital or institution, again to cover all its services. The difference between capitation and percentage of revenue is that the percentage of revenue may vary with the premium rate charged and the actual revenue collected, whereas capitation is a fixed amount of reimbursement—it remains the same regardless of how much or how little the HMO collects in premium revenue.

In both methods, the hospital or institution stands the entire risk for the cost of any services that it provides for the defined membership base; if the hospital cannot provide the services itself, the cost for such care is deducted from the capitation payment. For this type of arrangement to be successful, a hospital must know that it will be serving a clearly defined segment of an HMO's enrolled population and that it will be able to provide most of the services that those members will need. In these plans, the PCP is clearly associated with just one hospital. Alternatively, if the HMO is dealing with a multihospital system with multiple facilities in the HMO's service area, it may be reasonable to expect that the hospitals in the system can care for the HMO's members on an exclusive basis.

It is necessary to clearly define what is covered under the capitation plan and what is not covered. For example, the capitation plan may include outpatient procedures, but the HMO and hospital need to account for outpatient procedures that are performed outside the hospital's service area. Will home health care be part of the capitation plan, and if so, what agency is to provide that service? It is unwise to place the hospital at risk for services that it cannot control.

Capitation dramatically improves cash flow to the hospital (because it is prepayment for services), makes revenue predictable, and results in profits if utilization is well managed. In the recent past, however, some hospitals have simply not been able to manage the financial risk associated with capitation plans because they lack the financial management tools and expertise, utilization management skills, and information management capabilities necessary to manage the risks associated with a broad population of members. When the membership base of capitated lives is small, then chance becomes as important as clinical management, or even more so. As a result, many hospitals that once sought out capitation are now declining to participate in capitation programs. Overall, hospital capitation is not as common as it once was, and percentage of premium is now very rare.

Contact capitation, like that for physicians as described earlier, is also possible for hospitals. In the case of hospitals, the total monthly capitation amount is paid out to hospitals based on what percentage of total admissions for that month went to each particular hospital. Contact capitation can also be mixed with other forms of reimbursement, such as using case rates for obstetrics and excluding that service from the capitation program. Like in physician programs, contact capitation is theoretically attractive but difficult to administer fairly, and it is used rarely now, if at all.

Periodic Interim Payments and Cash Advances

It was once common but now is rare for an MCO to make periodic interim payments (PIPs) or a cash advance to a hospital to cover expected claims. A PIP is a regular cash payment made to the hospital, with actual expenses being deducted from the PIP on an ongoing (e.g., monthly) basis; the cash advance is similar but may not be quite as regular. The cash advance is periodically replenished if it falls below a certain amount. Hospitals may receive payment for services provided directly from the cash advance, or the MCO may pay claims outside it, in which case the cash advance serves as an advance deposit. The value of this approach to a hospital is that it ensures a positive cash flow. In fact, PIPs and cash advances are so valuable to a hospital that they may generate a discount by themselves.

This mechanism is particularly effective in those periods when an unusually high number of claims is overwhelming an MCO's payment system, or the MCO is otherwise unable to process payments in a timely manner. The cash advance allows the MCO to meet timely payment provisions and keeps the hospital financially sound while allowing additional time for the MCO to resolve problems with its payment systems.

Refusal to Pay for Serious Errors or Internal Inefficiencies

In any reimbursement method that is based on charges and/or days in the hospital, many MCOs refuse to pay for services that are incurred because of serious hospital errors or inefficiencies. For example, if a patient is admitted for a routine surgical procedure but surgery is delayed because of scheduling problems, the MCO will not pay for the extra day. Similarly, if a patient is admitted on a weekend and the hospital is unable to perform certain necessary diagnostic tests (e.g., the radiology specialty procedures unit is not open on weekends), the MCO will not pay for the weekend days that the patient spends in the hospital.

More serious are medical errors—sometimes referred to as "never events" because they are events that should never happen to a patient in the hospital—that cause serious illness or injury. In 2002, the National Quality Forum defined 27 such "never events" in six categories: "Surgical events (e.g., surgery being performed on the wrong patient or wrong body part), product or device events (e.g., using contaminated drugs), patient protection events (e.g., an infant discharged to the wrong person), care management events (e.g., a serious medication error), environmental events (e.g., electric shock or burn), and criminal events (e.g., sexual assault of a patient)." The MCO would not pay any costs associated with such "never events," and indeed the hospital should not charge for them. This list is expected to expand in the future.

Emergency Department

Except in some cases of capitation, how the MCO reimburses the hospital for inpatient services will differ from how it reimburses for emergency department (ED; formerly called the emergency room or ER) services. Methodologies for reimbursing for ED services are similar to those discussed next for outpatient procedures, although ED reimbursement and elective outpatient procedure reimbursement may be dealt with differently from each other. However, it is common for MCOs to require greater cost sharing by members for ED services unless the patient is admitted to the hospital, and there may be little or no coverage if it is determined that the ED visit was unnecessary (though that has become less common under pressures from regulators and legislators). In the event that a patient is admitted, the cost of the ED care may or may not be included in how the hospital is reimbursed for inpatient care, depending on what has been negotiated.

Unlike other services, hospitals have a legal requirement regarding emergency services. In 1986, the federal government passed the Emergency Medical Treatment and Active Labor Act (EMTALA) to prevent transfer or "dumping" of uninsured patients by private hospitals to public hospitals. EMTALA requires that all patients presenting to any hospital ED must have a medical screening exam performed by qualified personnel, usually the emergency physician. The medical screening exam cannot be delayed for insurance reasons, either to obtain insurance information or to obtain preauthorization for examination. Although theoretically an MCO could deny payment even though the ED was required by law to provide services, hospitals rightly refused to agree to those terms.

Outpatient Procedures

As care has shifted from inpatient to outpatient, so have charges, and outpatient charges can exceed the cost of an inpatient day. There are several ways that outpatient services for procedures are reimbursed, and they almost always differ from how inpatient care is paid. Charge-based reimbursement for outpatient procedures occurs more often than does charge-based inpatient care.

Discounts on Charges

Either straight discounts or sliding scale discounts may be applied to outpatient charges. Some hospital administrators argue that the cost of delivering highly technical outpatient care actually is greater than the average per diem cost of inpatient care, primarily because the per diem cost is based on more than a single day in the hospital, which spreads the costs over a greater number of reimbursable days. Some MCOs negotiate a clause in their contracts with hospitals to ensure that the cost of outpatient surgery never exceeds the cost of an inpatient day, whereas other MCOs concede the problem of front-loading (i.e., for an inpatient stay, all the costs occur right up front; the lower costs of the recovery days balance out the higher cost of the first day when the procedure occurred) surgical services and agree to pay outpatient charges at a fixed percentage of the per diem (e.g., 125 percent of the average per diem).

Package Pricing or Bundled Charges

With package pricing or bundled charges for outpatient procedures, MCOs bundle all the various charges (e.g., the cost of supplies, the room where the procedure took place, medications, nursing support, recovery room costs, discharge activities, and so forth) into one single charge. They may use their own data to develop the bundled charges or use outside data, such as those available from a national actuarial firm. Bundled charges are generally tied to a principal procedure code used by the facility. Bundled charges may be added together in the event that more than one procedure is performed, although the second procedure is discounted because the patient was already in the facility and using services.

Related to the use of bundled charges is the establishment of tiered rates. In this approach, the outpatient department categorizes all procedures into several categories. The MCO then pays a different rate for each category, but that rate covers all services performed in the outpatient department, and only one category is used at a time (i.e., the hospital cannot add several categories together for a single patient encounter).

Ambulatory Visits

In the reimbursement of ambulatory visits or encounters, there are two classification systems: ambulatory patient groups (APGs) and ambulatory payment classifications (APCs). Both are in the public domain. A variety of payers (e.g., Medicaid and several Blue Cross/Blue Shield plans) were using APGs prior to the introduction of APCs. Beginning in 2000, CMS began implementing APCs for outpatient prospective payment in hospital outpatient departments and ambulatory surgery centers for Medicare patients. Because of this, APCs are fast becoming the package pricing system of choice for MCOs.

Although APGs and APCs are based on procedures rather than simply on diagnoses, contain a greater degree of adjustment for severity, and are considerably more complex, they are to outpatient services what DRGs are to inpatient services. If more than one procedure is performed, the MCO will receive claims for each, but there is significant discounting for the additional charges.

Pay for Performance

Pay-for-performance, in which at least some portion of financial incentives is aligned with the practice of evidence-based clinical care, continues to grow. P4P programs began in HMOs, but regional and national companies are now using them in PPOs. CMS demonstration programs for use in FFS Medicare will further accelerate adoption beyond the HMO model. Unfortunately, with the exception of California, the programs currently in place vary from one another—an issue that creates difficulty for providers required to report data in multiple programs.

There is some overlap between P4P programs focused on hospitals and those focused on physicians, at least in regard to the clinical conditions under review, but the actual measures tend to be different. P4P programs for hospitals measure results for individual hospitals or health systems, whereas physician programs usually look at the performance of groups because there are usually only a small number of measures that any individual physician may be able to report. The exception to this is Medicare, in which process measures (e.g., did the physician write the prescription, even if the patient didn't fill it) for individual physicians are being instituted.

P4P programs are dependent on a variety of data collection approaches, which can lead to inaccuracies if not managed properly. Payers in several markets have come under pressure from regulators as well as threatened lawsuits around these programs, particularly when the data are used to tier networks, so leading payers maintain openness to improvements in methodologies for data collection.

Studies are appearing that either bolster or diminish the use of P4P. In fact, both proponents and detractors of P4P often cite the same studies to make their arguments. Despite the firm assertions of those directly affected, the effect of P4P remains unclear. Nevertheless, most of the leading payers, as well as many large employers and CMS, are committed to P4P, and programs continue to evolve.

Data Transparency

Data transparency, making information about cost and quality available to consumers, continues to increase. As with P4P, approaches to making such data available vary from one program to the next. In addition to demands for greater information by employers, a presidential order requiring any company or organization contracting with the federal government in health care to comply with transparency requirements has lent further impetus to such initiatives.

Commercial health plans, some state governments, and Medicare provide information to consumers in a dizzying array of formats. Cost comparisons may be based on average charges or contractual terms, may be averaged for all providers or individualized for others, and may be displayed using numerals or symbols. Quality measures, similar to those used in P4P, may be reported using symbols (e.g., three stars), a roll-up score (e.g., a single number), or roll-up scores for identified measures (e.g., a single number reflecting those measures associated with one clinical condition), and may be averaged or individualized. There are now efforts under way to standardize how data are collected from providers and provided to consumers, but at the time of publication, such standardization had not taken place.

There is even less known about the effectiveness of data transparency initiatives than for P4P. Some nonscientific surveys do demonstrate that at least some consumers may be using this information, but its overall effect on cost or quality may depend less on consumer behavior than on the "sentinel effect" (i.e., people changing their behavior when they know they are being observed). The simple fact of payers or governments looking at selected measures may be sufficient for providers to improve performance.

ANCILLARY SERVICES

Medical services provided as an adjunct to basic primary or specialty services are called ancillary services and include almost everything other than institutional services (although institutions can provide ancillary services). Ancillary services may be diagnostic or therapeutic. Ancillary diagnostic services include laboratory, radiology, nuclear testing, computed tomography (CT) scanning, magnetic resonance imaging (MRI) scanning, positron emission tomography (PET) scanning, electroencephalography, cardiac testing, and many other diagnostic interventions using advanced technology. Ancillary therapeutic services include cardiac rehabilitation, noncardiac rehabilitation, physical therapy, occupational therapy, speech therapy, and other forms of therapy that usually (but not always) require several visits.

Pharmacy services are ancillary services that account for significant costs and have been subject to price and usage inflation for many years. An MCO may consider mental health and substance abuse services to be ancillary, but they are really core services, though they will be discussed in this section. Emergency services, occasionally considered ancillary as well, are also actually core medical services and were addressed earlier.

Because most ancillary services require an order from a physician, the cost of such services is dependent on the utilization patterns of physicians. To reduce the cost of ancillary services, it is necessary to change these patterns (see Chapter 4). Many non-HMO MCOs also increase the amount of cost sharing by the patient to discourage demand for overuse. But the primary method of controlling the cost of ancillary services is to contract for such services in a way that makes the cost predictable. In fact, many MCOs rely far more heavily on favorable contracting terms to manage the cost of these services than they do on managing utilization.

Contracting and Reimbursement for Diagnostic and Therapeutic Ancillary Services

The development of a contracting and reimbursement system for ancillary services is one of the first and most important steps that an MCO can take in dealing with costs in this area. Many ancillary services are among the first to be carved out of the main medical delivery system and assigned to another organization able to achieve economies of scale and manage overall cost, quality, and service standards. HMOs will commonly also look for organizations that are able to accept the financial risk of providing such services and adhere to quality and service standards.

Closed-panel HMOs, large medical groups, and IDSs have the option of providing certain ancillary services in-house. Management must conduct a cost-benefit analysis to determine whether that is a better course of action than contracting with an outside provider. Managing utilization must still be undertaken even when the service is in-house, however, because there is often a perception that referral for that service is free and certainly convenient.

Open-panel and closed-panel MCOs that do not have ancillary services in-house must contract for the services. An MCO usually has its choice of hospital-based services (sometimes these are the only option), freestanding (independent) services, or office-based services. A combination of such factors as quality, cost, access, service (e.g., turnaround time for testing), and convenience for members determines the choice. Unlike the physicians who provide medical services, the set of providers of a particular ancillary service usually makes up a small percentage of the total number of providers. This allows the MCO to have greater leverage in negotiating with these providers and greater control over the quality of the services themselves.

In HMOs (or in rare non-HMO MCOs) that have absolute limitations on benefits for ancillary services, capitation is very effective. To establish a capitated reimbursement system for ancillary services, it is necessary to calculate the expected frequency of need for the service and the expected or desired cost, and then spread this amount over the membership base on a monthly basis. POS plans that allow significant benefits for out-of-network may still use capitation, but only for the in-network costs; they must pay out-of-network costs through the regular fee allowances. If the capitated provider limits access strictly or cannot meet demand, the MCO will end up paying twice—once through capitation and a second time through FFS. If the MCO has a large membership base, it may be possible to forecast cost and usage even under a POS plan, but if the MCO has a small enrollment base, capitation for benefit plans other than a pure HMO plan may not be feasible. This is because with a small enrollment base, the effects of random chance (e.g., the number of severe auto accidents) is higher than the effect of valid statistics (e.g., the number of auto accidents that can be expected for every 500,000 people).

Though this would be unusual, a non-HMO MCO may have no out-of-network benefits for some ancillary services, making it easier to establish a capitation system (i.e., because the MCO does not cover certain specific out-of-network ancillary services, it does not need to try and adjust for in-network versus out-of-network differences in cost). Simple PPOs generally are unable to use capitation because they are unable to adjust for in-network uses versus out-of-network use for any specific provider and must depend on fee allowances or other forms of episode-related reimbursement.

Not all types of ancillary services lend themselves to capitation. If an ancillary service is highly self-contained, it is easier to capitate; for example, physical therapy usually is limited to treatment given by physical therapists and does not involve other types of ancillary service providers. Home health care, on the other hand, often involves home health care nurses and clinical aides, durable medical equipment, home infusion and medication supplies and equipment, home physical therapy, and so forth.

A number of MCOs have successfully used capitation for home health care services, although those have tended to be larger MCOs with sufficient volume to permit the accurate prediction of costs in all these different areas. Other MCOs have been able to use this approach successfully only for parts of home health care (e.g., home respiratory therapy). In other areas, a combination of capitation and fixed case rates (e.g., for a course of chemotherapy) may be successful.

A variant on capitation that is similar to the single specialty management organization or specialty network manager discussed earlier may be used occasionally. In this case, a single entity accepts capitation from the HMO for all the providers of a particular ancillary service (e.g., physical therapy). That organization then serves as a network manager or even as an IPA. The participating ancillary service providers may be subcontractors to the network manager and may receive payment either through subcapitation or through a form of FFS. In all events, the network manager is at risk for the total costs of the capitated service even though the participating ancillary service providers are usually at risk as well through capitation, fee adjustments, withholds, and so forth.

MCOs that do not have the option of capitation, which are most MCOs, can still achieve considerable savings from discounts. Diagnostic ancillary services are often high-volume services, so it is usually not difficult to obtain reasonable discounts or to negotiate a fee schedule. Therapeutic ancillary service providers may be willing to accept case rates or tiered case rates. In this form of reimbursement, the ancillary service provider receives a fixed amount for a particular case regardless of the number of visits or resources used in providing services. For home health care involving high-intensity services such as chemotherapy or other high-technology services, the MCO may pay different rates depending on the complexity of the individual case. These types of reimbursement systems are often quite difficult to administer, requiring both the MCO and the provider to keep records manually.

When a limited number of providers are offering the ancillary service, it is more difficult to obtain substantial discounts and savings. Other than some types of exotic testing and therapy, this is usually not the case unless the MCO is located in a rural area. In general, good contracting makes it possible to achieve very high savings.

Contracting and Reimbursement for Pharmacy Services

Because they constitute a significant percentage of the total cost of health care, pharmacy services are especially important to managed care. In the past, the rate of inflation for pharmacy benefits was substantially higher than for any other single component of the health care dollar. Pharmacy costs are now closer in their inflation rate to most other types of services, though not for "specialty pharmacy," as discussed later in this section. The ongoing inflation in the cost of drug benefits is the result of increases both in the cost of drugs and in the total amount of drugs prescribed (Figure 3–5).

There are a few nontraditional methods of pharmacy reimbursement, such as capitation, but in general, these have not been successful. The forces that have led to increasing drug costs have made it very difficult to predict and manage the risk for drug costs. Therefore, most pharmacies will not accept such risk, and pharmacy benefits management companies are reluctant to do so either.

Traditional Pharmacy

The advent of new and more effective drugs has led to an increase in the use of drug therapy. New drugs are available to replace problematic older drugs in the treatment

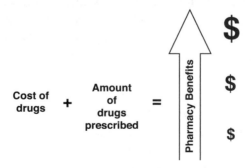

FIGURE 3–5 Factors Causing Pharmacy Benefit Cost Inflation

of such conditions as high cholesterol and high blood pressure—conditions that lead to silent diseases, so called because they have no obvious symptoms until the damage is severe (e.g., heart attack or stroke). Although the conditions had no symptoms, early drug treatments sometimes had side effects (e.g., niacin, administered for high cholesterol, causes flushing and heat flashes). Thus, many patients chose not to take any medication at all. With new drugs free of side effects, treatment became widespread.

In other instances, new drugs have been created where there was no alternative at all, such as the current "viral cocktail" regimens for the treatment of acquired immunodeficiency syndrome (AIDS). New developments in existing classes of drugs, such as antidepressants, have increased usage as physicians and patients search for the most effective drug in each case. Direct-to-consumer advertising by drug manufacturers also heightened demand for certain drugs. The introduction of so-called lifestyle drugs, such as pharmaceutical treatments for sexual dysfunction, has increased demand. Finally, the creation of so-called cosmeceuticals (i.e., drugs for cosmetic effects), such as those for hair loss or skin rejuvenation, has increased demand, though MCOs usually decline to cover costs for drugs in this last group.

Because new drugs are under patent and their production is monopolized, they tend to be priced high. The combination of the steep climb in the overall use of drugs and the expensiveness of drugs has made drug costs difficult to control. In recent times, many drugs that formerly were under patent have come off, and generic substitutions are available. By aggressively using benefits differentials, plans have been able to increase the use of generic drugs, which has slowed the excessive inflation rate. However, drugs that remain on patent also remain very expensive.

To aid in managing drug costs, virtually all MCOs use the services of a pharmacy benefits management company (PBM). In some cases, the MCO actually owns the PBM; in other cases, it is a freestanding company. As the name suggests, such a company specializes in managing drug benefits. The PBM processes the claims for drugs submitted by the participating pharmacies, manages the formulary (i.e., the list of approved or recommended drugs), and monitors utilization. The MCO and PBM work together to contract for a network of pharmacies, including a mail order pharmacy, to provide the drug benefits for the MCO members. It is common for the PBM to contract with national drugstore chains because only the largest companies can usually provide the favorable pricing required under its contract with the MCO. Because the PBM contracts with multiple chains, geographic coverage is usually very good, and even merely good geographic coverage is considered acceptable in return for the cost controls available through preferential pricing.

The usual method of reimbursing pharmacies combines a fill-fee and the ingredient cost. The fill-fee is an amount that the pharmacy benefits management company pays the pharmacy simply for filling a prescription regardless of the drug prescribed. For example, a pharmacy benefits management company may pay a pharmacy two dollars for each prescription filled. The ingredient cost is the cost of the drug itself. It is not easy to determine the ingredient cost because the price that a pharmacy pays a drug manufacturer may not be the same as another pharmacy. For example, nationwide chains are able to obtain lower prices (through their wholesale distributors) than small community pharmacies can obtain. It is common for the PBM to refer to a standardized listing of drug prices and to reimburse based on that standard, often referred to as the average wholesale price (AWP). The PBM commonly reimburses based on a percentage of AWP (e.g., 95 percent).

PBMs and MCOs (at least large ones) frequently negotiate a rebate from drug manufacturers. This approach does not apply to every drug, of course, but to drugs that are relatively common and for which multiple good alternative therapies exist. For example, if there are 15 different nonsteroidal anti-inflammatory drugs (NSAIDs), the PBM and the MCO may negotiate with the manufacturers of one or two of them to obtain rebates based on the inclusion of those drugs in the MCO's formulary. Inclusion in the formulary in this case represents preferential pricing, and the formulary will provide some type of indication that preferential pricing is in effect. Because of pressures following a federal lawsuit over how savings from rebates are applied, rebates are not as common as they once were.

Specialty Pharmacy

Specialty pharmacy is anything not on the standard formulary and that requires physician intervention/distribution, including a particular type of biopharmaceutical: proteins created via recombinant DNA replication that require injection either by a provider or by the patient. These drugs are used for uncommon conditions, for more common illnesses such as certain types of cancers, and for inflammatory diseases such as eczema and rheumatoid arthritis. Treatment ranges from expensive to enormously expensive; in some cases, treatment can exceed a quarter million dollars per treated patient annually. Although specialty pharmacy currently constitutes a relatively modest percentage of overall health care spending, it is rapidly becoming a major factor in cost inflation.

The management of specialty pharmacy is substantially different from that taken for traditional pharmacy. A traditional PBM or MCO may have a specialty pharmacy unit or may use a freestanding specialty PBM. Movement away from an AWP model and toward an average sales price (ASP) model more closely aligns pricing with acquisition costs. In this model, the MCO, PBM, or specialty PBM establishes a price for each specialty drug based on its ability to obtain a discount through direct purchase. Alternatively, the ASP is based on the average price that the manufacturer sells the drug for. The PBM or MCO then will reimburse providers of the drug based on that price, plus a modest percentage increase such as 6 percent, and no more. This eliminates the very high mark-up charge that providers routinely add for giving the drug (these drugs usually require adminis-tration by medical personnel). Some MCOs will also have a preferred vendor that will obtain and administer the specialty drug if another provider declines to ac-cept that reimbursement.

Biopharmaceuticals often come from only one or two manufacturers that are able to bypass the usual distribution channels, and retail pharmacies are not in-volved, making it difficult to obtain favorable pricing on certain specialty drugs. Payers use a combination of strict precertification to ensure proper indicated use, step therapy using less costly drugs first, and negotiating with manufacturers to try to contain costs in this area. But with more and more new biopharmaceuti-cals in the development pipeline, most payers see this as a substantial source of cost inflation.

Contracting and Reimbursement for Behavioral Health Services

It is very common for MCOs to carve mental health and substance abuse services out when contracting for a medical care network. Because the management of be-havioral health services is substantially different from the management of any other type of medical care, MCO medical managers turn to specialty organiza-tions. These services are often referred to as mental health and substance abuse (MH/SA) services but will be referred to here as behavioral health services.

Often, an MCO contracts with a specialized managed behavioral health or-ganization (MBHO) to build the behavioral health services network, reimburse the providers, and manage the cost and quality of the services provided. The MBHO may be a company, or it may be a behavioral health specialty group or facility. In other cases, especially if the MCO is large enough, it may have the in-ternal capabilities to manage behavioral health networks and services.

If the MCO is an HMO or HMO-like, it might pay for behavioral health ser-vices through capitation. In other words, it might pay a specified amount per member to the behavioral health services organization, which then assumes full management of behavioral health services. The organization does not necessarily pay the actual service professionals through capitation, however. Like the arrangements with IPAs discussed earlier, the behavioral health services organization accepts financial risk but may pay the professionals on a different basis, such as FFS or salary.

It is common for the network of behavioral health service providers to include substantially fewer than the total universe of available providers. In the case of behavioral health services, the size and scope of the network is particularly complex because there are so many different types of service providers: psychiatrists, psychologists, therapists with a master's degree (e.g., master of social work [MSW]), therapists without a master's degree (e.g., licensed clinical social worker [LCSW]), and various types of substance abuse therapists. The MBHO usually determines the number and types of therapists that the network needs to provide adequate access and then contracts accordingly. Reimbursement of professionals, therefore, is usually on a FFS basis, though capitation sometimes does occur when a large professional group takes on responsibility for all behavioral health services.

NETWORK MAINTENANCE AND MANAGEMENT

It is not enough to build a network. As noted earlier, there are many ongoing activities required of an MCO to maintain and manage the network. Recredentialing is an example of a common and required network maintenance activity. Related to this is the measurement and management of the performance of the network.

Access to care is the first and most important issue that an MCO faces. The MCO must ensure that the network is large enough and covers the proper geographic area to allow the MCO membership good access to all health care services. This means monitoring the number and types of provider practices by geographic location (usually ZIP code) and the number of practices actually open to members of the MCO in each location. For example, the MCO may be experiencing a high level of growth in a particular section of its service area, and the network management may need to recruit new providers in that area. Or the MCO may appear to have sufficient numbers of providers in an area, but many of those practices may be closed to new members (i.e., the providers are not accepting new patients). In this case, the MCO network management must recruit new providers and work with existing providers to see if they can or will open up their practices to new patients.

Individual providers, especially physicians, benefit from individual attention. The drug companies know this well, which is why they send sales representatives to visit physicians on an individual basis. Similarly, many MCOs require their network management departments to visit each provider at least once or twice a year, although the largest national health insurance companies find this to be too expensive. More attention may be paid in the case of providers who have specific issues. For example, some providers will have complex billing issues, or problems accessing member eligibility information; in such cases, additional time spent by network management staff may prevent further problems. Orientation of new providers and reorientation of existing providers to the way that the MCO operates are also individual-based activities.

On the less pleasant side, the MCO must occasionally deal with providers who are performing poorly, either financially or clinically (e.g., by providing substandard medical care or inadequate access to services). In each case, the MCO must either help the provider improve in the relevant areas or take action to remove the provider from the network. The termination of a contract with a provider, as noted earlier, is not easy to carry out and is likely to involve complex legal and regulatory issues. Fortunately, such actions are only rarely necessary.

CONCLUSION

An MCO's network of providers is its vehicle for providing health care to its members at an affordable cost. The composition of the network is directly dependent on the type of benefits plans being administered and has a direct bearing on the MCO's ability to manage the cost and quality of the care provided. Contractual terms between the providers and the MCO are a hallmark of managed care, and many of the provisions of such contracts are regulated. The maintenance of a network requires just as much work as does the original creation of the network. Reimbursement of providers is an integral part of the overall management of utilization and quality of clinical services, but all provider payment systems are tools, not ends in themselves. Like all tools, reimbursement systems are useful only in the context of the other tools being used. Managing quality and utilization effectively is essential for achieving positive results; reimbursement schemes alone will never be enough.

NOTE

1. Federal Register 45 C.F.R. Part 60.

CHAPTER 4

Management of Medical Utilization and Quality

LEARNING OBJECTIVES

- Understand the basic components of utilization management
- Understand the different approaches to managing wellness and prevention, basic medical services, ancillary services, chronic diseases, and case management
- Understand the nature of external review
- Understand the basic components of quality management

The term "managed care" derives from the practice of managing certain aspects of the delivery of medical services, focusing in particular on cost and quality. Cost, to oversimplify, is the result of two variables: price and volume. Chapter 3 briefly describes the price part of the equation (i.e., the reimbursement that providers receive). This chapter describes the volume part (i.e., the utilization of medical services). The terms "utilization management" (UM) and "care management" (CM) refer to the practice of managing medical services utilization; the term "UM" will be the one used in this chapter to avoid confusion. Although technically a function of UM, the specialized functions of disease management (DM) and case management (also abbreviated as CM) are considered separately.

Managed care organizations (MCOs) typically attempt to manage the quality of medical services as well. For some types of MCOs, such as health maintenance organizations (HMOs), quality management (QM) is required by law or regulation. A strong QM program can also be demanded by large employers or by accreditation programs such as those described in Chapter 7. Recently, accreditation agencies have also developed QM standards for preferred provider organizations (PPOs), though PPOs with a strong QM program still remain the exception and not the rule.

The privacy requirements of the Health Insurance Portability and Accountability Act (HIPAA; see Chapter 7) and various state privacy laws set limitations on access to medical information for purposes of UM and QM. For instance, only that medical information required to correctly authorize or pay for services can be used. In other words, the UM and QM functions of an MCO cannot simply "go fishing" in any individual's health records. If the information is "de-identified" (i.e., stripped of any information that could allow it to be traced to an individual), then there are generally no restrictions on its use.

Members of an MCO are asked to give consent to having their medical information reviewed and are provided with plain language forms to help them understand why it is being reviewed. Although the consent process can be cumbersome, it serves to protect patient confidentiality. In the event that a member refuses to allow the MCO's medical management function to access his or her medical information, the MCO may reduce the benefits paid for services (the difference in coverage would be described in the member's description of benefits). Such consent documents are routinely provided when an individual signs up for a health plan, as well as from a provider prior to treatment (when possible) and on claims forms. Special consent may be required for some UM or QM activities related to behavioral health.

THE USE OF BENEFITS DESIGN TO CONTROL COST

Before discussing medical management, it is worth briefly addressing the use of benefits design in controlling costs. Prior to managed health care, health insurance companies relied almost solely on cost-sharing with members to try and control cost, with the exception of service plans (see Chapter 2) that also had contracts in place with providers. As discussed in Chapter 1, the advent of HMOs reduced cost-sharing dramatically, replacing it with medical management. The idea was to provide more benefits—including benefits that had not been previously provided, such as prevention and drug coverage—and to pay for it by reducing spending on care that was medically unnecessary or not cost-effective. As the market pushed back through the "managed care backlash" described in Chapter 1, cost-sharing was reintroduced in MCOs. To be accurate, it had never completely gone away, but in recent years, it has become a significant factor in MCOs' strategies for managing costs.

Benefits are now being designed to not only require members to share a greater portion of overall costs but also to provide both incentives and disincentives for certain types of care. For example, it is common for MCOs to have little or even no cost-sharing for prevention (discussed next) but to have increasing amounts of cost-sharing for increasingly costly services. Requiring higher copays or coinsurance (see Chapter 2) for care received from a subspecialist or surgeon rather than a primary care physician (PCP) is now common, as are high levels of cost-sharing for expensive testing or treatment. However, an MCO may waive cost-sharing in certain circumstances—for example, not requiring cost-sharing for something that helps a patient to stay out of the hospital. In general, the less an MCO actively manages care, the more it relies on benefits design to control costs.

Prevention and Wellness

Dr. Paul Elwood coined the term "health maintenance organization" to highlight the idea that HMOs were dedicated to providing preventive services. Indeed, although such services were not covered by most health insurance policies prior to the spread of HMOs, they have since become the norm.

Preventive services, unsurprisingly, are aimed at preventing certain diseases. Childhood immunizations are the most common type of preventive care, but prevention also includes other services such as adult immunizations, Pap smears, mammography, and screening for high cholesterol, high blood pressure, diabetes, and other common chronic diseases. Wellness programs are directed at helping members to change their lifestyles and develop healthy habits. Weight loss programs are now routinely emphasized, as are smoking cessation, exercise, and various other "healthy lifestyle" programs. Not every MCO provides a full range of wellness programs, but they have been steadily increasing in popularity.

Health risk appraisals (HRAs) are an overall assessment of a new patient's medical condition and risk factors. Automated feedback based on responses to an HRA serves to encourage a member to make better health choices. Examples of such feedback might include the value in potential added "life-years" from losing weight or stopping smoking, or the value in having routine screening tests done.

In managed care, HRAs are also designed to uncover information on member issues requiring intervention by the MCO to preserve health and lower overall costs. Different types of HRAs may also be focused on specific groups of members, such as commercial, Medicare, or Medicaid members. Many advanced Medicare HMOs, in doing an HRA, go well beyond data-gathering forms and physical exams and actually send a nurse or home aide to the residence of a new member. During the visit, the nurse or aide may do a nutritional assessment, check for compliance with prescribed medications, and look for simple interventions that could save problems later, such as providing an inexpensive bathmat to prevent the member from slipping in the tub and breaking a hip.

Basic Utilization Management

Basic UM usually refers to those routine functions that an MCO applies to manage the cost of the most common medical services. Basic UM is considered distinct from DM and CM, which are discussed in the next section. Basic UM encompasses prospective, concurrent, and retrospective activities (Figure 4–1). Prospective activities are intended to influence utilization before the fact, concurrent activities are intended to influence utilization as it occurs, and retrospective activities include reviewing utilization patterns to determine where improvements need to be made.

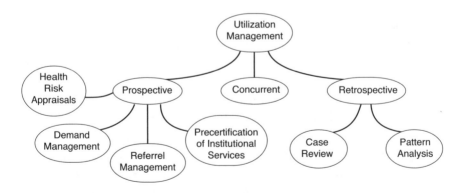

FIGURE 4–1 Components of Utilization Management

Measuring Utilization

Many different types of measurements are used when managing utilization. Utilization is almost always measured using a standard set of calculations, and depending on the type of MCO, those measures may be refined even more. In many cases, something is measured as per member per month (PMPM) or per member per year (PMPY). For example, physician encounters (i.e., visits to physicians) in a commercial (non-Medicare/Medicaid) HMO may be reported as 3.4 visits PMPY, meaning that on average, members saw a physician 3.4 times per year. Or, utilization costs for a particular type of service may be reported as $10.15 PMPM, meaning that on average, that service costs the MCO $10.15 each month for each member.

Another common form of measurement is per thousand. This measurement is usually for units of service, but is sometimes (though not commonly) used for cost as well. For example, most plans measure bed days per 1,000 plan members (sometimes abbreviated as BD/K). Measurements per thousand may be used for any time period but are most commonly used on a monthly or a yearly basis. For example, a commercial HMO may report 220 BD/K for the month, meaning that for every 1,000 members, an average of 220 hospital days were used each day of that month; it may also report that for the entire year, utilization was 231 BD/K, meaning that over the course of the entire year, for each 1,000 members, an average of 231 hospital days were used each day. Closely related are admissions per thousand, and average length of stay (ALOS).

Prospective Utilization Management

Prospective utilization management includes demand management, referral management, and precertification of institutional services.

Demand Management

Demand management is intended to influence the future demand for medical services. The most common demand management methods include providing access to preventive services, convenient hours of operation, and medical advice manuals for use at home. Many MCOs also provide a more active method: providing a round-the-clock nurse advice line so that members can access a trained nurse 24 hours a day, 7 days a week by calling a toll-free number. The advice lines rely heavily on clinical protocols. Many MCOs that have advice lines have seen a decline in the use of their emergency departments.

Referral Management

Referral management, sometimes referred to as referral authorization, is principally confined to HMOs that use the so-called gatekeeper model. In this model, a member's PCP determines which medical services are truly necessary, coordinates the provision of these services, and thereby discourages overuse of services. The provision of care by any health care professional other than the PCP must be authorized by the PCP. (Note that virtually all MCOs also offer coverage allowing women to have direct access to obstetricians and gynecologists.)

The authorization requirement allows the PCP to determine if a health problem or condition requires treatment by a specialist. If it does, the PCP authorizes a referral to a specialist under contract to the MCO. The authorization is seldom open ended. It is usually for a limited number of visits (e.g., one to three) except in defined circumstances (e.g., chemotherapy is fully authorized for the entire course of treatment).

It is rare for an MCO to become involved in the authorization process other than to capture the authorization data to process the claim properly. The PCP is expected to exercise proper clinical judgment without the MCO's intervention. The MCO should provide the PCP with periodic reports containing data on referral rates and costs, as well as reports on the PCP's capitation pool or withhold if that is appropriate (see Chapter 3 for a discussion of capitation and withholds).

Precertification of Institutional Services

Prospective management of institutional services, both inpatient and outpatient, is a staple of managed care in all types of MCOs. It is also referred to as precertification. The process is simple: someone calls the MCO to request authorization for an elective admission or outpatient procedure, the MCO checks the request against clinical criteria and whether the facility is in the contracted network, and the MCO authorizes the procedure or not. In the case of an inpatient admission, the MCO usually assigns an expected length of stay (LOS, or less commonly, ELOS) as well.

Clinical criteria for authorization are commercially available, but the MCO may have developed its own criteria. Likewise, maximum allowable LOS guidelines are commercially available, but the MCO may modify those guidelines to suit the local area. Most MCOs are now using computerized programs to determine quickly whether the clinical criteria are met and to capture pertinent data.

Who calls the MCO for authorization depends on the type of health benefits plan. For indemnity insurance plans or for the out-of-network benefits in PPOs and POS plans, the member must call or face an economic penalty. For HMOs and the in-network benefits in POS and most PPOs plans, the burden of responsibility is on the provider, and it is the provider who suffers an economic penalty for failure to comply.

The economic penalties vary based on the type of health benefits plan. If authorization is obtained before the admission or procedure takes place, there is no penalty. If authorization is not obtained, a penalty will be imposed. In some cases, the penalty is noncoverage (e.g., this would be the penalty in an HMO with no out-of-plan benefits). In a PPO or a POS plan, the penalty may be a higher level of coinsurance (e.g., 50 percent of the cost of the service). In an emergency situation, a penalty is not imposed as long as the MCO is notified within a reasonable period of time (usually one business day after the admission).

Concurrent Utilization Management

Concurrent review of utilization, also known as continued stay review, applies almost exclusively to inpatient care and to complex, expensive cases. Most MCOs, such as service plans, PPOs, or large HMOs with numerous network hospitals, will typically perform a concurrent review from a remote site via telephone. The MCO's UM nurse will call the hospital to ascertain the status of the case. If the case is on track, no further action is taken. If the hospital stay is going to exceed the previously authorized days, the UM nurse will collect clinical data and either authorize the additional days or deny coverage for them. Rather than deny coverage, however, the UM nurse is far more likely to work with the physician and the hospital's own utilization review and discharge planning department to facilitate the patient's discharge. For example, home physical therapy or outpatient treatments may be arranged.

HMOs that more actively manage utilization will often send a UM nurse to the hospital to obtain more detailed and timely information and more actively manage the case. The process is otherwise the same as just described, but communications and information exchange are better than when only the telephone is used. Some large organized medical groups may use a hospitalist (a physician who only attends inpatient cases; see Chapter 3) as well.

In the event of ambiguity or disagreement during the concurrent review process, the UM nurse refers the case to a physician working with or for the MCO (either the medical director or a physician adviser). This physician may call the attending physician to discuss the case and may then make a determination regarding authorization for further payments. If the attending physician and the medical director cannot agree on the need for, or the appropriateness of, the care, an external review process may be used, as described later in this chapter.

Retrospective Utilization Management

Retrospective utilization management activities fall into two broad categories: case review and pattern analysis.

Case Review

In case review, past cases are examined for appropriateness of care, billing errors, or other problems. If an error or irregularity is found in a particular case, the MCO may adjust payment or at least investigate the case. If there is some suspicion that a provider is chronically making errors or even committing fraud, the MCO may place the provider on regular review.

In almost all instances, the case review process is routine, and any problems discovered are the result of simple errors by providers. The vast majority of providers would never engage in fraud, but there is always the possibility that a few will, and the MCO must be on the alert for cheating. If fraud is detected, the MCO must determine whether the case is serious enough to warrant notifying the authorities or instead try to deal with the provider by itself—by demanding that the money be returned, for example, and then removing the provider from the network. In more serious cases and in cases involving Medicare, the MCO must notify law enforcement agencies as well as a Federal data repository.

Pattern Analysis

Pattern analysis involves the amassing of significant amounts of utilization data to determine if patterns exist. These patterns may be provider specific (e.g., over- or underutilization of certain tests or procedures) or planwide (e.g., an unanticipated increase in cardiac testing costs). After a pattern has been found, the reasons for it must be investigated so that corrective action may be taken.

MCOs continually seek to improve how they provide retrospective data to the network providers to allow the providers to compare themselves with their peers and modify their own practices as appropriate. This form of feedback promises to be a powerful additional tool for controlling health care costs and quality. It is also directly related to efforts in data transparency programs in which MCOs provide comparative data about cost and quality to members.

External Review of Coverage Decisions

Most MCOs are required to provide for external review of disputed coverage decisions (this process is also discussed in Chapter 7 because similar appeals processes are usually required under state and federal laws). In the review process, outside specialists (i.e., specialty physicians who do not work for the MCO) look at the relevant facts of a particular decision to determine whether the MCO should provide coverage for medical services for which it has denied coverage. External reviews, though available to all members, are not common, and when they occur, they typically involve treatments that are experimental or would generally be considered medically unnecessary.

Here's how the review process might come into play. Suppose that a member of an MCO has a continuing severe medical condition and that the attending physician recommends a risky or experimental procedure, such as an unusual type of transplant. Given the likely assumption that the MCO's benefits policy excludes coverage for experimental or unproven procedures, the MCO may decide that this procedure falls into the unproven category and deny coverage. The attending physician, however, might dispute that the procedure is actually experimental and argue instead that it should be covered. If the medical director of the MCO continues to deny coverage, the member (often through his or her physician) could request an external review. The MCO then would contact a panel of specialists who are in the same specialty as the attending physician but do not work for the MCO (other than doing external reviews), and, with the consent of the member, it would provide these external reviewers with relevant medical information. The member and the attending physician would also provide whatever information they wish to the panel. The panel may hold a hearing or discuss the case with the attending physician and the medical director, but whatever the process, it will eventually issue a determination as to whether the MCO is liable for coverage of the procedure. That decision is then binding upon the MCO.

External review programs are required in 44 states and the District of Columbia as of 2007. Under a federal law called the Employee Retirement Income Security Act (ERISA), there are also appeal standards that apply even to self-funded health plans that are not otherwise subject to state laws. ERISA provides standards for how, and how quickly, a member may appeal a denial of coverage, including a right to have medical judgment aspects reviewed by a neutral third-party specialist, though the exact requirements are usually somewhat different from those found in most state laws. Although one might think that appeals would generally be granted, the denial of coverage is upheld about as often as it is overturned.

Disease and Case Management

Disease management and case management focus on conditions that are chronic, expensive to treat, or both (Table 4–1). It is no surprise to anyone that a small percentage of members of an MCO account for a very large percentage of the MCO's total medical costs. Although the majority of members have routine medical needs, some have serious chronic medical conditions—for example, severe diabetes, acquired immunodeficiency syndrome (AIDS), or certain heart conditions—that require a great deal of expensive medical care. Likewise, certain acute cases—such as a severe automobile accident or a very premature newborn—are also expensive.

The related functions of large case management and disease management are designed to address the medical needs of members requiring very expensive care. By paying particular attention to these members, the MCO is able to lower costs while improving outcomes and quality. It is common for MCOs to use outside companies to conduct their DM activities because a large company that focuses only on DM is better able to stay current with advances in treatment options and make the necessary investments in information technology (IT) to support these specialized clinical functions. It is less common for MCOs to outsource CM, but that occurs as well. A few MCOs conduct all these activities using internal resources.

Case Management

Case management of catastrophic or chronic cases, whose costs often exceed routine costs by several orders of magnitude, has the potential to deliver substantial savings. In this type of utilization management, trained nurses coordinate aspects of care, such as rehabilitation, home care, health education, and the like, and thereby improve outcomes as well as reduce expenses.

Disease Management

Disease management is a special form of case management in which the MCO focuses on a handful of selected diseases and works proactively with each patient to control the disease's course. The usual result is greater continuity and a better outcome. Much attention is directed toward trying to make the patient's condition better through different approaches or at least preventing it from getting worse. The hallmark of a disease management program is the inclusion of numerous types of health professionals, not just physicians. For example, a clinical pharmacist may play a more active role in treating childhood asthma than the pediatrician (e.g., by teaching the child how to use inhaled steroids). Likewise, a dietitian may be of great service to patients with a severe heart condition by teaching them how to maintain a good diet and avoid unhealthy habits.

Table 4–1 Comparison of Conventional Case Management and Disease Management

Traditional/Catastrophic Case Management	Disease Management
Emphasis is on single patient	Emphasis is on population with a chronic illness
Early identification of people with acute catastrophic conditions (known high cost or known diagnoses that lead to high cost in the near term)	Early identification of all people with targeted chronic diseases (20–40) whether mild, moderate, or severe
Acuity level of catastrophic cases are high, acuity level of traditional cases are high to moderate	Acuity level is moderate
Applies to 0.5–1% of commercial membership	Applies to 15–25% of commercial membership
Value relies heavily on price negotiations and benefit flexing	Value due to member and provider behavior change that results in improved health status
Requires plan design manipulation	Requires no need to change plan design
Primary objective is to arrange for care using the least restrictive clinically appropriate alternatives	Primary objective is to avoid hospitalization *and* modify risk factors, lifestyle, and medication adherence to improve health status
Episode is 60–90 days	Intervention is 365 days for most conditions
Site of interaction primarily hospital, hospice, subacute facility, or home health care	Site of interaction includes work, school, home
Driven by need for arrangement of support services, community resources, transportation	Driven by nonadherence to medical regimens
Outcome metrics are single-admit LOS and cost per case	Outcome metrics are annual cost per diseased member and disease-specific functional status

Source: Adapted from D. W. Plocher, "Fundamentals and Core Competencies of Disease Management," in *The Essentials of Managed Health Care,* 5th edition, ed. P. R. Kongstvedt (Sudbury, MA: Jones & Bartlett Publishers, 2007), 238, table 10-1.

Identification of Candidates for Case Management or Disease Management

An MCO or a company performing DM and/or CM for an MCO must have multiple ways of identifying which members might be good candidates for CM or DM. Individuals with clinical conditions who would benefit from greater interventions may be identified by nurses or hospitals during utilization review, through computer programs that analyze claims for diagnoses and for the types of drugs being prescribed, through abnormal laboratory results, through HRAs, or through using sophisticated modeling programs to try and predict which members may be deteriorating clinically. In addition to identifying these members, it is important to determine just what level of intervention would be most appropriate. This process is illustrated in Figure 4–2.

Ancillary Services

Ancillary services, described in Chapter 3, are medical services that are not personally provided by physicians and are not hospital or institutional services. The two common types are diagnostic services and therapeutic services. As noted in Chapter 3, examples of ancillary diagnostic services include laboratory, radiology, nuclear testing, computed tomography (CT), magnetic resonance imaging (MRI), electroencephalography, and cardiac testing. Examples of ancillary therapeutic services include cardiac rehabilitation, noncardiac rehabilitation, physical therapy, occupational therapy, and speech therapy (but not behavioral health services, which are discussed later in this chapter).

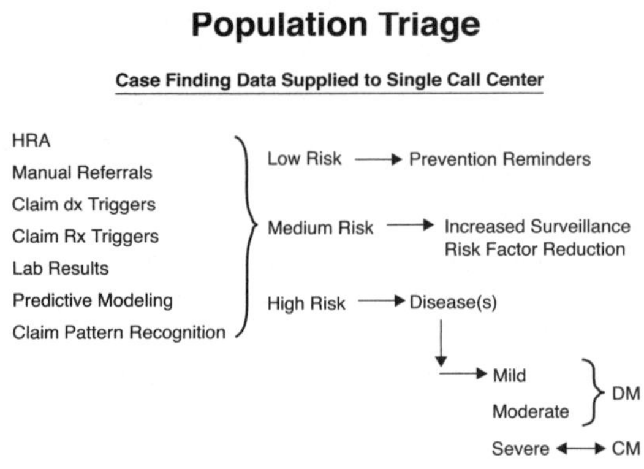

Population Triage

Case Finding Data Supplied to Single Call Center

HRA
Manual Referrals
Claim dx Triggers   Low Risk ——▶ Prevention Reminders
Claim Rx Triggers   Medium Risk —▶ Increased Surveillance
Lab Results   Risk Factor Reduction
Predictive Modeling   High Risk ——▶ Disease(s)
Claim Pattern Recognition

Mild   } DM
Moderate }
Severe ◀—▶ CM

FIGURE 4–2 Identification of Candidates for Case Management or Disease Management

Active management of ancillary diagnostic and therapeutic utilization is usually done only by those MCOs that actively manage most aspects of care, such as an HMO. Active management makes use of several approaches (Figure 4–3). First, excessive ordering of ancillary services by some physicians can often be reduced through practice profiling and feedback, as well as direct discussions between the medical director and these physicians.

Another strategy is to limit the number and duration of certain types of ancillary services that can be authorized at once, at least on a routine basis. For example, an MCO may allow only 3 weeks of routine physical therapy services to be authorized initially; if additional weeks of therapy are needed, they would require an additional authorization. The restriction on the original authorization forces the physician to reassess the case and determine whether the services are still useful.

For a small number of expensive services not commonly used, the MCO may put into place precertification using standards of care. Before ordering an expensive test, for example, a physician might have to suspect a particular diagnosis (one that the test pertains to) rather than order the test just to see what turns up.

Many MCOs, particularly non-HMO plans, do not actively manage utilization of ancillary services. Rather, they depend on benefits design, cost-sharing, and favorable contracting to address costs. Although favorable contracting has already been discussed in Chapter 3, it is such a cornerstone of controlling costs of ancillary services that it bears mentioning here. Capitation is well suited to ancillary services in HMOs and some POS plans, but favorable contracting can deliver substantial savings for any type of MCO. The basic principle is to develop ancillary service provider–MCO contracts according to which the providers charge the

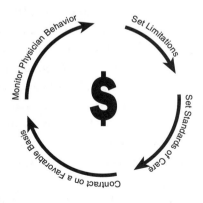

FIGURE 4–3 Methods for Managing Ancillary Service Costs

MCO reduced fees in return for being part of a restricted network and getting referrals from the MCO. The contracts should include quality and service requirements that providers must meet and should offer the providers financial incentives for meeting these requirements.

Pharmaceutical Services

Drug benefits are handled differently than other types of health care benefits such as hospital or physician care. Until managed care became prevalent, prescription drugs, like preventive care services, were not even covered by insurance. Now it is rare for an MCO not to provide coverage for drugs, although the benefits differ from plan to plan. The cost of drugs accounts for a large part of the health care dollar—around 12–15 percent of total health care costs for the typical MCO. Pharmaceutical services are further divided into standard or routine pharmacy and specialty pharmacy.

Management of Routine Pharmacy Services

In prior years, the rate of inflation for drugs was much higher than in any other area of health care because of the high cost of patented "blockbuster" drugs. In addition to the cost of individual drugs, far more drugs are being prescribed than ever before. Many new drugs have been developed in the past 10 years, and physicians can now treat certain conditions far more effectively with these drugs than previously. But the growing use of treatment with drugs comes at a price, because new drugs are generally expensive. Recently however, so many brand-name drugs have come off patent, allowing any drug maker meeting certain standards to make and market them as the generic equivalent of the brand-name drug, that the rate of inflation for drugs is about the same as for most other types of care.

Many MCOs contract with an outside organization to manage their pharmacy benefits (Exhibit 4–1). Organizations of this type are commonly called pharmacy benefits management companies (PBMs). PBMs rarely assume financial risk for drug costs but are responsible for all aspects of management. A PBM will typically contract with many MCOs to grow large enough to achieve economies of scale and negotiate better financial terms (see Chapter 3). The largest MCOs may actually own their own PBM, though even then, the PBM is managed as a separate company.

In managing drug benefits for an MCO, a PBM makes use of the following elements, as well as other less important ones.

EXHIBIT 4-1

Why Managed Care Organizations Use Pharmacy Benefits Management Companies

Formulary. A PBM may negotiate discounted rates with manufacturers of certain drugs listed in the formulary.

Drug utilization review (DUR). Contract allows PBM or MCO to manage volume and nature of prescriptions as well as provide special authorization for certain drugs.

Benefits design. Contract provides for lower costs when members resort to less expensive alternatives.

Mail order. Mail order provides for less expensive costs in filling prescriptions for chronic medications.

Formulary

A formulary is a list of drugs covering typical medical needs, although it does not include all the available drugs for each medical condition. In many cases, several drugs are equally useful for a particular condition but differ widely in price. In addition, the PBM, because of its size, may have negotiated volume discounts with the manufactures of some of those drugs. The formulary, then, contains drugs that are effective and are the least costly among the alternatives. If one particular drug is clearly the most effective, that drug may be the one listed on the formulary regardless of cost.

The PBM provides the MCO with a formulary, which is then modified by the MCO's pharmacy and therapeutics (P&T) committee to meet the needs of the network physicians. For example, the P&T committee may determine that a drug not on the formulary really needs to be included and will ensure that it is. More often, the P&T committee reviews requests for exceptions, such as for highly expensive and infrequently used drugs for which the indications for use are not always clear.

The use of multiple tiers within a formulary is almost universal in MCOs and is discussed in the Benefits Design section in this section of the chapter.

Drug Utilization Review

Drug utilization review (DUR) consists of activities and strategies for managing the volume and pattern of prescriptions. The most common DUR strategy is to create prescribing profiles and provide the profile information to the physicians so that they can compare their prescribing patterns with those of their peers.

Another common strategy is to require special authorization for certain drugs. Authorization requirements are usually restricted to a very small list of drugs that have the potential for being prescribed inappropriately. This approach is most commonly used for specialty pharmacy drugs as discussed in a moment.

Benefits Design

Though not technically a utilization management function, the design of prescription drug benefits is an important element of the overall approach. One simple strategy for affecting utilization is to charge members a lower copayment for using less expensive alternatives. This is accomplished through the use of a tiered formulary.

Tiering stratifies drugs according to how much the member will share in the cost. For example, generic drugs may be classified as Tier 1, and the member has only a $10 copay. Certain brand-name drugs that are effective and for which the MCO has favorable payment terms may be classified as Tier 2, and the member has only a $20 copay. Expensive brand-name drugs for which there is a good Tier 1 or 2 alternative may be classified as Tier 3, and the member has a $50 copay. Some MCOs even use a fourth tier for drugs for which coverage is very limited but not zero. In all cases, the pharmacies under contract to the PBM are supposed to provide information to members about alternatives to the most expensive drugs.

Benefits may also be limited to a certain amount of a drug. For example, drugs for erectile dysfunction in men are often limited to 7–10 per month. Other drugs used strictly for cosmetic purposes, such as drugs for baldness in men, may not be covered at all.

Mail Order

All PBMs provide a mail order service. Members may be required to use mail order for any chronic medications—that is, drugs that are always used by the member, such as blood pressure medicine. Mail order is never used for acute prescriptions that are limited as to how long the patient will take the drug. Typically in mail order, a 3-month supply of the drug is dispensed at a time. Mail order lowers the fill-fee (i.e., the payment to a pharmacy to fill the prescription) and allows for greater discounts by purchasing drugs in bulk from the manufacturers.

Management of Specialty Pharmacy Services

Specialty pharmacy is anything not on the standard formulary, and most important, a particular type of biopharmaceutical: specialized manufactured proteins requiring injection either by a provider or by the patient (but not including insulin). These drugs are used both for uncommon genetic illnesses and some more common ill-nesses, such as certain types of cancers and certain inflammatory diseases like eczema and rheumatoid arthritis. Treatment ranges from expensive to enormously expen-sive; in some cases, treatment can exceed a quarter million dollars annually per treated patient. Although currently a relatively modest percentage of overall health care spending, specialty pharmacy, with more and more new biopharmaceuticals in the development pipeline, is rapidly becoming a major factor in cost inflation.

The management of specialty pharmacy is different from that used for phar-macy in general, so it may be managed by the MCO's PBM, or it may be man-aged by a PBM that focuses only on specialty pharmacy. Biopharmaceuticals for a specific clinical condition often come from only one or two manufacturers who bypass the usual distribution channels, and pharmacies are not involved. MCOs use a combination of strict precertification to ensure proper indicated use, DUR and step therapy using less costly drugs first, and negotiating with manufacturers to try to contain costs in this area.

MCOs have also been changing how they pay for specialty pharmacy, following Medicare's lead. These MCOs establish a price for each specialty drug based on the MCO's ability to obtain a discount through direct purchase, or else on what the manufacturer sells the drug for to the providers that administer it. The MCO then will reimburse the provider based on that price plus a set administration fee (e.g., 6 percent of the cost of the drug, and no more). This dramatically reduces the very high profit margin that is typically built in when a provider administers these drugs.

Finally, in the past, benefits for coverage of injectable drugs were included under the major medical policy (i.e., treated like benefits for hospital services, not like a drug benefit). MCOs are increasingly moving specialty pharmacy to the drug benefit portion of the policy, providing for the same types of tiering and cost-sharing used for routine drug coverage.

Behavioral Health Services

Behavioral health (BH) services, which includes both mental health and sub-stance abuse therapy, are also unique, and most MCOs take different approaches to managing it. In reality, although these services were once closely managed by MCOs, and HMOs in particular, it has become more common to use benefits de-sign to place greater cost-sharing on members who seek BH services. Contracting for favorable rates is also commonly used. HMOs may capitate an external or-ganization as discussed in Chapter 3, and that organization is then responsible for managing cost and access. Even MCOs that do not capitate frequently contract with specialized BH management companies because traditional UM is not generally appropriate for BH.

Outpatient BH is usually managed via telephone calls between trained clinical reviewers discussing cases with patient's therapists, or increasingly via data transmission or secure forms using the Internet. The management of inpatient care, being more expensive, uses precertification and concurrent review tailored for BH. More important, a BH management program places greater emphasis on reducing the need for readmission by looking at improving ambulatory care follow-up, using community resources, and, when appropriate, involving an employee assistance program that many employers make available.

Quality Management

MCOs vary in their approach to medical QM. Indemnity and service plans and even PPOs generally are less aggressive in managing quality than are HMOs, although, like all generalizations, there are notable exceptions. As in UM, as MCO model types progress through the continuum, greater attention is paid to managing quality, and more resources are expended on this task.

As discussed in Chapter 7, there are external accreditation agencies that verify whether an MCO is meeting standards for measuring and improving quality. External accreditation of quality programs was once confined only to HMOs, but in recent years, these agencies have developed standards for PPOs and other types of MCOs. The results of certain quality measures are often published by these agencies as well, the most well known of which is the Health Care Effectiveness Data and Information Set (HEDIS). Another common set of measures is called the Consumer Assessment of Healthcare Providers and Systems (CAHPS). CAHPS was begun by the federal government for use in Medicare and Medicaid managed care plans but is now used alongside HEDIS in commercial plans as well. Maintained by a federal agency, its focus is now expanding beyond MCOs to ambulatory providers, hospitals, and the Medicare prescription drug program.

Quality has also become a higher priority for providers. That is not to say that providers ignored quality in the past, but in 1999, the Institute of Medicine's Committee on the Quality of Health Care in America published *To Err is Human: Building a Safer Health System*, followed in 2001 by *Crossing the Quality Chasm*. These two publications described both deficiencies in quality and patient safety in our health care system, and what steps to take to change that. The committee proposed six aims for improvement in our health care system: care should be safe, effective, patient centered, timely, efficient, and equitable (specifically meaning that all people should get the same level of quality care). These concepts are incorporated in most MCOs' QM programs.

Almost all MCOs begin the quality management process by verifying the credentials of participating providers (see Chapter 3). Beyond credential verification, MCOs generally employ two approaches to quality management, often together: classic quality management and total quality management (or continuous quality improvement). Following is a brief description of these approaches.

Classic Quality Management

The classic approach to managing quality is based on the works of Avedis Donabedian.[1] The three key elements are structure, process, and outcome (Figure 4–4).

Structure. The task here is to look at how the infrastructure of the MCO is related to quality and to make changes in the infrastructure to bring about quality improvements. Structure studies might, for instance, examine medical records (e.g., to verify the presence of a drug allergies list or review laboratory notes), immunization records, access to care (e.g., the length of time between calling to make a routine or urgent appointment and the appointment date), waiting times in the office, telephone responsiveness, and so forth. These studies may be done on-site by the MCO's quality management nurses or self-reported by a provider.

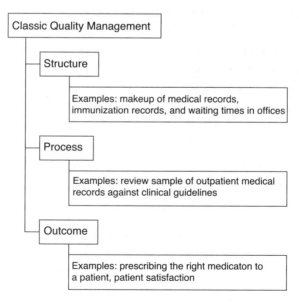

FIGURE 4–4 Classic Quality Management

A special type of structure study examines the effect of the utilization system on access to care. In particular, the MCO gathers data to discover whether utilization is inappropriately low and whether the authorization system is acting as a barrier to necessary care.

Process. The care process is the way in which care is actually rendered. To investigate the care process, MCO nurses typically review a sample of outpatient medical records in light of the clinical guidelines established by the quality management committee using published evidence-based medical practice guidelines. Clinical guidelines are specific to a particular disease or procedure. For example, guidelines on the diagnosis and treatment of ear infections are common and typically include the steps of the history and physical exam that a physician should record, and the appropriate types of treatment and follow-up that should occur. Guidelines are also common for inpatient care, such as for the diagnosis and treatment of heart attacks (early detection and aggressive treatment of heart attacks have been shown to be beneficial, as has the use of beta blockers after discharge). After reviewing the medical records and/or measuring compliance with clinical guidelines, the MCO reports back to the providers. These reports note deficiencies and clearly state what corrective actions need to be taken. Conditions that are routinely examined include cardiac diseases, asthma, chronic lung diseases, diabetes, and similar common chronic illnesses.

By way of example, in the past, despite the known usefulness of beta blockers, many patients who had heart attacks were discharged from the hospital without being placed on these drugs. Most major MCOs now provide feedback to physicians who are not prescribing beta blockers and indicate that their prescription is the standard of practice (unless there is a good medical reason countering their use, such as the presence of congestive heart failure). Now, compliance with this practice is high. For any process measured, after a suitable period of time has passed, the MCO will conduct an identical study to ensure that appropriate changes in practice behavior have occurred. For inpatient care, the MCO may rely on the hospital's own quality management program to report results, with only random external audits by the MCO.

Large MCOs have begun to automate the review of process. Using claims data on discharge diagnoses, outpatient claims diagnoses, and drug claims diagnoses, these plans are employing sophisticated computer analyses to determine whether patients are receiving appropriate prescriptions, such as in the beta blocker example. These automated programs are not foolproof, however. For example, a system looking to see if a physician is checking for protein in the urine of a diabetic patient (a routine type of test) may not detect that the test is being done if the physician does not submit a separate claim for using a simple dipstick test rather than sending the patient for a more expensive lab test. Continued improvements in automated systems should begin to address such shortfalls.

Outcome. In evaluating the outcome of care, MCOs generally look at adverse events and MCO-wide measures. One particular set of adverse events are known as "never events," which are 28 serious and costly errors in the provision of health care services that should never happen, such as amputation of the wrong limb, leaving a gauze pad in the abdomen following surgery, or a serious fall by an ambulatory patient. Following the lead of Medicare, MCOs are looking to put in place policies of not paying for costs associated with never events. Another distressing common adverse event is the prescribing or dispensing of the wrong drug, which has recently been recognized as more common than previously imagined; it too is considered a never event if it leads to a serious complication. It must be noted that providers themselves, especially hospital systems, are well aware of the pervasiveness of medical errors and are working independently to prevent them.

An MCO will perform outcomes studies to uncover whether its providers are generally successful at treating designated conditions. It might, for example, look at the rate for control of hypertension without preventable side effects, the rate for delivery of healthy babies, and so forth. The MCO will choose conditions that occur often enough to measure and then determine what represents a good outcome. Defining a good outcome is not as easy as it seems because many conditions cannot be cured, only controlled. The quality management committee is responsible for choosing what types of outcomes to measure and how to determine if an outcome is successful. Desired outcomes may also differ depending on the type of plan, with some differences between commercial plans, Medicare, and Medicaid groups.

If the rate of successful outcomes for a given condition is not acceptable, the MCO quality management function may study that condition further, using structure and process studies as well. An example will serve to illustrate how these studies can work together. Suppose the MCO chooses to look at the outcomes of cardiac bypass surgery. The study discovers high success rates except at one hospital. The MCO then analyzes the data and finds that patients who have surgery at that hospital end up going back to surgery (i.e., being operated on a second time) much more often than do patients who have surgery at other hospitals. The MCO and/or the hospital then conducts a process study, which uncovers the fact that the hospital's standards of care for postoperative care (i.e., care given immediately after surgery) do not contain the same infection control procedures found in other hospitals, or worse yet, the procedures exist but are not being followed. At this point, there may be enough information for the hospital (and the physicians, of course) to change what they are doing to correct the problem. But to take the example in a slightly different direction, suppose that a structure study shows that the machine used for sterilizing certain instruments is not being serviced properly. The incorrect servicing and the difference in infection control requirements together would be considered the likely causes of the postoperative infections and the lower success rate for cardiac bypass surgery experienced by the one hospital.

Member satisfaction is among the outcomes that an MCO might study. The MCO will typically survey members regularly, analyze complaints, and so forth, to determine overall satisfaction levels and to act on identified problems. As noted earlier, as well as in Chapter 7, the most common satisfaction survey in use is CAHPS, though many MCOs supplement this with their own specific surveys.

Total Quality Management

Managed care has adopted many of the tenets of the approach to industrial quality improvement referred to as total quality management (TQM) or continuous quality improvement (CQI). This approach makes most sense for closed-panel MCOs, but all types of MCOs can benefit from TQM/CQI techniques. Although these techniques can be quite complex, the basic strategy is simple—to continually reexamine what is done and how it is done, with the goal of doing it better. In other words, the strategy is to not stop with good enough but to strive continually to do better.

Whereas the classical approach to quality management focuses on conforming to standards, TQM and CQI emphasize the importance of improving the standards. These two approaches are not inconsistent. The only way to know if the medical care provided by an MCO conforms to the current best practices is to document these practices and measure the care provided against them. But practices change, and the goal of TQM/CQI is to search out new best practices and ensure that medical care changes to conform to these.

The medical practices that MCOs address tend to be different from the ones that health researchers address. For instance, health researchers at a teaching hospital may perform rigorous clinical studies to determine which of two clinical protocols (i.e., ways to deliver care) is better. These studies are commonly used to evaluate treatments for cancer, AIDS, and so forth. MCOs may participate in such studies but are rarely their primary sponsors. Instead, MCOs focus their quality improvement efforts on issues directly under their control. Common examples include finding better ways to notify members about needed preventive care (e.g., immunizations and mammograms), better ways to identify drug interactions, and better ways to help patients recover faster following surgery.

Finally, many MCOs apply TQM/CQI techniques to their overall operations. By doing so, they seek to lower administrative errors, increase administrative efficiencies, and lower administrative costs.

CONCLUSION

A handful of factors distinguish managed care from indemnity health insurance. The presence in managed care of a contracted network of providers and favorable pricing is one such differentiator. However, simply obtaining a better price for medical services, although necessary for controlling costs, is not by itself any indication that health care is being managed. It is the management of utilization and quality that truly sets managed care apart.

Utilization management and quality management are constantly evolving. What worked well 10–15 years ago is now less valuable and in some cases has even been abandoned. As MCOs and providers become more sophisticated in dealing with issues of overutilization and variable quality of care, managed care will change to take advantage of the improvements.

NOTE

1. A. Donabedian, *Explorations in Quality Assessment and Monitoring, Vol. 1: The Definition of Quality and Approaches to Its Assessment* (Ann Arbor, MI: Health Administration Press, 1980).

Internal Operations

For every dollar paid to a managed care organization (MCO), somewhere between 8 and 16 percent is spent on administrative activities or internal operations, and the rest is spent on medical care. The terms "administrative activities," "internal operations," and "administration" are used interchangeably to describe everything an MCO does because, other than group or staff model health maintenance organizations (HMOs), MCOs do not provide medical care. The management of medical cost and quality (discussed in Chapter 4) and the provider network (discussed in Chapter 3) are also considered to be administrative activities, though an MCO may occasionally delegate these functions (and the cost to do them) to some form of integrated delivery system (IDS).

Typically, most members' interactions with the MCO will be administrative in nature, whether the member is applying for an identification card or resolving a complex claim for medical services. Today's MCOs are highly complex organizations that are required to conduct a vast array of business processes, but for the purposes of this discussion, internal operations to be discussed include:

- Marketing and sales
- Enrollment and billing
- Claims administration
- Member services
- Finance and underwriting
- Information technology (IT)

Network and medical management, although considered administrative functions as already noted, were discussed in Chapters 3 and 4 and therefore will not be discussed further in this chapter.

Many administrative services may be seen as "middleman" services and viewed as adding little value. Indeed, during the mid-1990s, the term "middleman" was used as an insult, with providers and consumers alike tending to believe that administrative services were largely a waste of money. Consequently, many providers attempted to take over administrative functions themselves to "cut out the middleman." As noted in Chapter 2, almost all these attempts ended in disaster. Whatever the attitude of providers or consumers toward these services, there is no question that internal operations are complex, are specialized, and cannot be done poorly. Furthermore, whether a particular type of service actually adds value is subjective (i.e., the answer depends on who is considering the issue). For example, does a state or federal regulation requiring the creation of yet another report add value? To regulators, the answer might be a clear yes; to an MCO, the answer may be less apparent.

MARKETING AND SALES

There can be no MCO if there are no enrolled members. Therefore, the first critical operational activities an MCO must undertake are to market its services and sell its products. The terms "marketing" and "sales" are often used synonymously, although marketing is not quite the same as sales. Marketing involves creating a strategy for entering a market and building the infrastructure needed to sell the

MCO's services. Sales, on the other hand, is the actual activity of selling to those in a position to buy. Marketing and sales do not set prices, however; that is the responsibility of the actuarial and underwriting functions, which are discussed later in this chapter.

By way of illustration, the marketing department may determine that the MCO should target small employers in its service area. It would then identify these employers, the issues that might make the MCO attractive to them, the best approach to selling the MCO's products to them, and so forth. The marketing department is responsible for creating supporting material, such as brochures and descriptions of the MCO's offerings, as well as advertising, public relations, and other broad activities designed to increase the visibility and enhance the reputation of the MCO in the market. Marketing is also usually involved in the development of new products—a high-deductible health plan (HDHP) or consumer-directed health plan (CDHP), for example—in addition to the strategy for growth in that product line.

Sales personnel are responsible for contacting the employers and meeting with the benefits managers. Personal discussions with the benefits manager of an employer allows the MCO's sales representative to find out the employer's priorities when it comes to purchasing health care benefits for employees and to describe what the MCO offers that would be of value to the employer. The sales representative also discusses financial terms, guides the employer through various benefits design options, and so forth. In other words, all the activities that involve face-to-face dealing with customers are the domain of the sales staff.

In the small-group market, sales personnel may focus primarily on their relationships with brokers, as discussed in the next section. In the case of the individual market (products sold to individual consumers either directly or through brokers), sales personnel may work with brokers or may communicate directly with consumers. Finally, sales personnel are usually dedicated to only one or two market segments, as described later.

Distribution

Distribution refers to whom or how the MCOs products reach the market. There are a variety of different channels for distribution, and Figure 5–1 illustrates examples in the commercial (i.e., nongovernmental) marketplace.

The MCO's own sales personnel are individuals employed by the MCO to represent it in the marketplace. Sales personnel also work directly with brokers, agents,

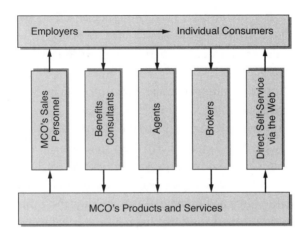

FIGURE 5-1 Distribution Channels

and consultants, though they usually focus on only one type. Individuals in sales are usually paid a relatively low base salary, supplemented by significant incentive payments for successful sales; the more they sell, the more they make. A similar compensation structure is often in place for individuals in marketing, but usually it is somewhat less weighted toward incentive payments. The more sophisticated MCOs look not only at sales and growth but at profitability as well in order to encourage profitable growth rather than growth that may not be profitable.

Benefits consultants are independent consulting firms that work directly for an employer. Consultants focus almost exclusively on large employers and receive a consulting fee from the employer that is not related to the premium cost of insurance and is paid on a one-time basis. Consultants do not need to be appointed or certified by an MCO because they are not representing the MCO in the market. Rather, consultants evaluate proposals from various MCOs against many criteria to help large employers make the best choices for employee benefits. Consultants also negotiate prices with an MCO on behalf of their clients.

For insured products, sales may be conducted by brokers or agents. Brokers are usually fully independent individuals or businesses that are licensed to sell the insurance products of many different companies. In return, they typically receive a percentage of the premium, a greater percentage for the initial sale, and then a smaller percentage of each month's premium collected from their clients (which is built into the cost of the premium). Brokers generally serve the small-group and individual markets (discussed next) but sometimes do represent large employers. In some markets, virtually all small-group business is sold through brokers. A broker cannot simply sell the product of an MCO, however, but must first be appointed or certified by the MCO. Agents are similar to brokers but may be affiliated with only one company or a small number of companies. Both brokers and agents usually sell insurance products for many services other than health—for example, life insurance.

Finally, it should be noted that many MCOs are supplementing their approach to sales by adding self-service options. This means that individuals, or even small companies, can apply for insurance via the Internet. They must answer several questions and may need to have medical screening, but the rest is fully automated, and sales personnel are not involved. In other cases, they can apply via the Web, but then a sales person does get involved in finalizing the sale. Such automated approaches are now being used by some larger agencies and broker companies as well.

Market Segmentation

As already noted, the market for managed care is not uniform, and it is important to understand the differences between the various segments. First, segmentation by organizational size is common in the commercial market. Large employers purchase services differently than small employers do, and midsized employers occupy, well, the middle ground. Therefore, it is common for the sales department of an MCO to organize its internal operations around segments based on organizational size. The sales department might also separately treat (1) national businesses with widely scattered locations, (2) local employers, and (3) individuals not covered through an employer (the individual purchaser market). Rules vary depending on whether an employer is purchasing insurance or is self-insuring (see Chapters 2 and 7 for discussion about self-insuring, sometimes called self-funding); sales of insured products must follow rules set out by the state, whereas sales of self-funded products follow rules set out by the federal government. Further commercial market segmentation often exists, even within each broad category, but a more detailed discussion of the topic is not warranted here.

MCOs that serve the beneficiaries of government programs view those programs as segments. Medicare is (usually) an individual product, but one that requires special training and knowledge. Medicaid may be sold on an individual basis, or beneficiaries may be enrolled by state agencies. Health benefits offered to federal employees are also unique, though benefits offered to state and local governments are more like large employer accounts. How marketing and sales may be conducted for Medicare, Medicaid, and federal employees is subject to very strict rules, and failure to follow those rules can result in penalties to the MCO.

Wholesale versus Retail

The commercial and governmental markets may be thought of as having wholesale and retail components. The wholesale component consists of employers and government agencies, whereas the retail component consists of individual consumers (Figure 5–2). In most cases, an MCO will market and sell to both components.

Selling to the employer involves an agreement between the MCO and the employer to offer the MCO's products to the employer's employees. In other words, a commercial sale begins with a sale to a group (the wholesale), and it is this sale that allows the MCO's products and services to be offered to employees in the first place. Selling to a governmental agency is much more bureaucratic and involves the MCO demonstrating that it can meet strict requirements set out by the agency.

The retail aspect of sales varies. In a small group in which there is no option besides the MCO, retailing may not be done or may focus on those employees that choose not to have coverage at all. Most midsized and large employers give their employees the option of choosing a health benefits plan from one of several MCOs, however, and even when one MCO is used exclusively, an MCO may offer several different plan designs (e.g., a high-option plan and a low-option plan).

Medicare and Medicaid beneficiaries fall into many different categories, and MCOs that serve those markets usually do not serve all categories; for example, nursing home residents are in a different category than are low-income families, and similar differences exist in Medicare. Medicare is almost always strictly retail once the MCO is approved to sell products in that sector. In other words, the sales personnel or brokers authorized to sell to the appropriate categories of Medicare beneficiaries do so by signing up individual consumers. The relatively uncommon exception to this is when an employer offers a Medicare product to retirees and pays for some or all of the cost of the added benefits. In that case, it is treated more like a group for purposes of sales.

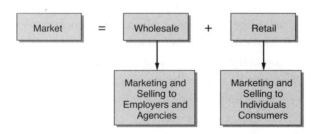

FIGURE 5–2 Wholesale versus Retail

Medicaid may or may not be retail, depending on the state. In some states, Medicaid-specific MCOs may be encouraged to sell to individual beneficiaries. More commonly, enrollment in Medicaid-specific MCOs is performed by the state Medicaid or social services agencies themselves. In some states, Medicaid beneficiaries in the appropriate categories are not given a choice, but are simply enrolled in the MCO.

Large Employer Groups

Large employers, roughly defined as employers having more than 2,000 employees, are usually self-insured (Exhibit 5–1). There is little agreement about when to start calling an employer a "large employer," and many in the industry would use

EXHIBIT 5–1

Market Size Segmentation and Characteristics

Small employer groups (2–50 covered lives)
The small-group segment represents the largest number of employer firms. Some MCOs further differentiate between very small (e.g., under 10 lives) from other employers in this segment. Some states allow a small business to have only one employee and still be treated as a group. Products are fully insured, and premium rates offered to the small-group segment are usually heavily regulated by the state. States usually do not allow premiums to vary based on experience.

Midsized employer groups (50–2,000 covered lives)
This segment may also be called the middle market. Some MCOs further differentiate between smaller groups (e.g., fewer than 250 lives) and other employers in this segment. As the employee size increases, these employers become more like large groups. Benefits may be less regulated, premiums may vary based on experience, and larger groups may self-insure.

Large employer groups (more than 2,000 lives)
The large employer generally has many worksites in multiple states and needs many different options. Benefits design varies much more, and premiums are either fully experience rated or, more commonly, self-insured.

1,000 or 3,000 employees to identify an employer as "large." Large employers often have sites in different geographic areas or even in different states. Large MCOs, particularly national companies, seek to offer large employers more than one benefits design—for example, both a health maintenance organization (HMO) and a preferred provider organization (PPO) design, or a PPO and a high-deductible health plan (HDHP). By offering multiple products, the MCO is able to avoid losing market share to a competitor that offers similar products.

Self-insured employers bear the financial risk for medical expenses themselves rather than purchasing insurance to protect against the financial risk. As noted elsewhere in this book, assuming the financial risk for medical expenses allows them to avoid paying state insurance premium taxes and also to avoid state-imposed requirements, such as mandated benefits, mandated inclusion of certain providers, and state-specific appeals and grievance programs (but not federal appeal rights). Even though they are self-insured, however, they also purchase stop-loss insurance, sometimes called reinsurance. This protects them from the cost of extremely expensive claims.

Large employers purchase health benefits for their employees primarily through consultants who specialize in employee benefits. This type of firm charges fees to the employer for its services and receives no income from the MCO as part of each sale. Because a self-insured employer is taking on the financial risk for medical expenses itself, it is primarily interested in an MCO's ability to administer the benefits program that it wishes to provide its employees. A benefits consulting firm helps to design the actual benefits package and then determines the requirements that an MCO must meet to administer this package. The cost of administrative services is subject to intense negotiation, with the employer wishing to pay as little as possible while demanding a high level of performance. Large employers commonly require any MCO they contract with to:

- provide adequate network access to care (defined by the number of available providers per geographic area),
- act in a timely fashion in paying claims, resolving problems or complaints, and so forth,
- be certified by a recognized accreditation agency (see Chapter 7), and
- offer medical management performance guarantees.

Despite the number of large employers that are self-insured, when an individual who has health benefits coverage from a large company sees a provider, the provider (and the member of the MCO, for that matter) typically assumes that, because the member is carrying an identification card with the MCO's name on it, the MCO is providing the insurance. But really it is the employer that is providing the insurance, determining the benefits package, and so forth, with the MCO administering the benefits plan on behalf of that employer. Even then, however, although there are likely to be differences in what is and is not considered a covered benefit when compared with the MCO's insured products, how the MCO pays claims and so forth will usually look the same to a provider.

Small Employer Groups

Small employers, roughly defined as having between 2 and 50 employees, occupy the opposite end of the spectrum. These employers are unable to afford the risk of self-insuring and therefore purchase group health benefits insurance from an MCO. A small employer usually has a single site or several sites in a restricted geographic area (exceptions occur, of course). It is unusual for a small employer to offer more than one type of health benefits plan or contract with more than one MCO because of underwriting risks associated with having more than one insurance carrier in a small account.

Some states allow businesses with only one employee to be considered a group. Health insurance offered through an employer is fully deductible from the taxes of the employer, unlike health insurance purchased by individuals in which there is limited, if any, deductibility. Benefits and rates in the small-group market are also heavily regulated, which can also mean that the cost is very high for a small business. HDHPs, with their lower costs, have been increasingly attractive to this price-sensitive segment. Even so, although most large and medium-sized employers offer health insurance, a significant percentage of small employers do not because of cost.

In the case of a small employer, the wholesale is really the entire sale, because the employees do not have multiple carriers to choose from. Of course, many employees have working spouses with access to a health benefits plan, and these employees can choose to forgo coverage and depend on the coverage of their spouses. In other cases, employees may choose to not take up coverage even though offered by the employer because of cost. For many MCOs, if the percentage of employees participating in the health plan falls too low (e.g., fewer than half), the MCO may decline to cover the employer; this may not be allowed in many states, however.

A small employer may purchase health benefits coverage directly from a sales person from the MCO or even directly via the Web, but usually a broker facilitates the sale. The broker helps the small employer find appropriate health benefits coverage, provides advice, and receives as ongoing revenue a percentage of the premium payment that the employer makes to the MCO.

Midsized Employer Groups

The dividing lines between small, medium, and large employers are, of course, arbitrary. At the extreme ends—that is, in the case of very small and very large employers—the ways that an MCO markets and sells services are definable. In the middle, things are less clear, although the larger an employer is, the greater the likelihood that it will use a consultant rather than a broker and will self-insure rather than purchase insurance. The transition to use of a consultant and to self-insuring occurs at no set point, but it frequently happens when an employer grows to be around 500 employees.

Individual Purchasers

Individuals purchase health insurance or managed care in fundamentally different ways than groups do. Medicare beneficiaries are individual purchasers of a sort, but the Medicare markets are so unusual that it is discussed separately in Chapter 6.

Individuals have much greater difficulty buying health insurance of any kind than do employee groups, for example. Their ability to acquire health insurance is affected by state laws and regulations and by the Health Insurance Portability and Accountability Act of 1996 (HIPAA; see Chapter 7), and in general, it is directly related to their age, sex, and existing medical conditions. This does not mean that an individual who is older or has an existing medical condition cannot purchase health insurance, although there are circumstances in which this is so.

Individuals who are younger and have no medical conditions that require ongoing care usually are able to purchase health insurance policies at reasonable rates.* The policies may exclude certain conditions, however. For example, individual policies commonly exclude pregnancy because of the risk that a woman will buy an insurance policy covering pregnancy services, get pregnant, make use of the covered services, and then drop the policy, preventing the insurance company or MCO from ever recovering the cost of the health care provided. Some states do not allow such exclusions, and in those states, the price of all individual policies must be raised substantially to pay for the services of those who use them and cancel their policies soon thereafter.

---

* Reasonable from the standpoint of the MCO, but not necessarily from the standpoint of a young and healthy consumer. Many such individuals choose not to pay high monthly insurance premiums when they rarely seek medical attention, and they must pay a high deductible when they do. This generally works out fine unless they get hit by a bus.

Not all MCOs or insurance companies offer individual policies for purchase in the open market. Those that do may be required to do so under state laws that mandate a so-called open enrollment period—a period in which each MCO must accept any person who applies for coverage. In a state where a mandated open enrollment period exists, individual policies typically are expensive and are not marketed or sold except as required by state law (e.g., the state may require the MCOs to advertise during defined periods and via defined types of notices). MCOs that actively market to individuals often do their sales through brokers, though many are now directly selling through the Web as well. An individual applying for coverage must pass underwriting criteria before a policy is issued (see the following section on underwriting).

There are many circumstances under which a person has the right to purchase an individual health insurance policy. For instance, if the person has recently lost coverage under a group policy (e.g., as a result of being laid off), he or she may have the right to purchase coverage from the MCO of his or her former employer, though only for a limited period. In other circumstances, if an individual is able to prove continuous coverage by another carrier, he or she has the right to purchase coverage from another carrier. This does not mean that the cost of the health policy will be low, however. Because the individual purchaser market is such that people can drop their health insurance policies whenever they want or not buy insurance in the first place (i.e., unlike in the case of auto insurance, no one is compelled by law to purchase health insurance), healthier and younger people tend not to buy individual health insurance policies, whereas older and less healthy people do. Therefore, the overall risk for medical costs tends to be higher than normal in most health plans in which people have a right to buy individual insurance policies. These rights are discussed further in Chapter 7.

Finally, the issue of providing health insurance to those who do not have it and cannot afford it or even get it is one that is the focus of a great deal of public policy debate. It is beyond the scope of this book to discuss the various approaches to decreasing the number of Americans without health insurance, but dramatic changes in federal or state approaches to this problem may directly affect some of what is discussed in this section.

Determining What to Sell

Every MCO offers multiple products, and the sales department must determine what products and services to sell to each employer. An employer may have a firm idea of what type of product it wants, but usually it will want to balance the various factors in making its purchasing decisions, and the sales staff will work with the employer to weigh these factors. The factors that an employer will consider in choosing a health benefits plan include the cost of the plan, the degree of coverage provided, the degree of access to network care, and the size of the network (Figure 5–3).

The MCO will have an array of standard products in each broad category (e.g., HMO, PPO, and HDHP). For each product type, most MCOs also have differing levels of copayment or coinsurance for office visits, different deductibles, different levels of drug coverage, and so forth. If the employer is a large one, it will, via its benefits consultants, typically create specialized benefits plans (e.g., plans that have special limitations on coverage for certain conditions). The sales staff, in conjunction with the underwriting staff, must work with the employer to determine the cost and feasibility of the options that the employer wishes to consider.

ENROLLMENT AND BILLING

Enrollment and billing are straightforward MCO functions. The enrollment and billing department ensures that new members are entered into the MCO's administrative IT systems, identification (ID) cards are generated and issued (by law, an MCO must issue such "evidence of coverage"), and so forth. Ongoing maintenance of membership eligibility files is also a critical function for a variety of reasons.

There are many circumstances under which a member's eligibility for health benefits must be verified. For instance, a hospital will want to confirm that a patient is covered under a health plan in order to properly bill the MCO or health insurer. If it is not possible for the hospital to verify eligibility (or if the patient is using an ID card for coverage that she or he no longer actually has), it will make other payment arrangements with the patient. Verification of eligibility is increasingly being done via automated self-service. Examples of these types of self-service include secure lookup functions via the Internet, secure direct communications between the IT systems of the MCO and a large provider system, interactive voice

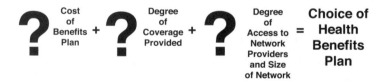

FIGURE 5–3 How to Choose a Health Plan

response via the telephone, and through the use of swipe-card technology (working with established credit card issuers) at the time of service.

Another example of the need for accuracy in the enrollment system concerns capitation in HMOs. Capitation payments are actually prepayments for services and should only be made for members who are actually covered by the MCO and whose premiums have been paid. If the MCO has not updated its membership database, it will incorrectly make capitation payments for former members and also will fail to pay providers proper capitation for recently joined members.

The MCO bills employers based on enrolled members. The seemingly simple activity of billing is actually quite complex and prone to error. In any company, employees are hired, and employees leave throughout the year. Also, qualifying "life events," such as marriage, birth, and adoption, may change the number of people covered under a policy. Thus, the membership database must be updated each month. However, updating is not always practical, especially in an MCO with thousands of employer customers.

In addition, employers are not always good about notifying MCOs about employment changes. Further, as might be expected, terminations constitute a far worse problem than new hires. New employees want their health coverage to become effective immediately, and thus they have a reason to go through enrollment, but employers sometimes have no formal process for disenrolling employees when they leave (voluntarily or not). Even employers that have a formal process do not always notify the MCO in a timely manner.

The drawbacks of carrying ineligible members as active members are obvious. First, the MCO may pay for health benefits services for individuals whose premium payments have not been received. Second, the MCO may pay capitation for such individuals. In addition, the MCO will believe that it is entitled to receive premium payments for such individuals and will book the revenue (though it has not received the cash) as accounts receivable, and correcting the mistake results in a negative revenue adjustment.

CLAIMS AND BENEFITS ADMINISTRATION

The claims department is responsible for ensuring that the providers are paid for their services and that members who have paid providers out-of-pocket receive the reimbursement that they are entitled to. In other words, at the most basic level, the claims department administers the health coverage benefits of the MCO. In the case of capitation, the finance department may pay the providers, but even then, the claims department will still process encounters (i.e., claims submitted by capitated providers that are counted for purposes of data capture but are not paid). However, as noted in Chapter 3, in all but a few MCOs (those that globally capitate IDSs), the vast majority of health care services generate claims that must be paid. The role of the claims department is consistently underappreciated by individuals who do not understand how an MCO operates.

The basic elements of claims processing are deceptively simple (Figure 5–4): Receive the claim (usually electronically, but also on paper), adjudicate (process) the claim using automated tools, correct errors that pop up the first time the claim is adjudicated and run them through again, adjudicate manually those claims that cannot be processed automatically, write a check, inform the member and provider what was paid and what was not, and finally, archive (store) all that information. What could be complex about that? Plenty. The claims functions affect and are affected by all other areas within the MCO (Figure 5–5). Although it is beyond the scope of this book to go into great detail, it is worth discussing the basic processes.

Claims Capture

The first function performed by the claims department is to capture the claim, which means entering a received claim into the claims processing system. Claims may come in from a variety of sources, but the most common sources are electronic submissions using nationally standardized electronic claims forms, and U.S. mail; less common sources are fax, secure e-mail, and self-entry via the Web (another form of standardized electronic claim, actually).

Claims usually come directly from the providers, but when a member receives care from a nonparticipating provider and pays for that care at the time of service, the subscriber (the member who has the coverage, regardless of whether the patient was the member or one of the member's dependents) will submit the claim.

Submitted claims must contain certain pieces of information, or they will be rejected by any MCO. Examples of such information include identification of the subscriber, who actually received the care, what care was received, when it was received, and so forth, all using specific types of codes. Electronic claims are standardized now under federal law, and no provider may submit a nonstandard type of electronic claim. Paper claims often use standard forms as well. Any claim that does not meet minimal data or informational requirements will be rejected at this point and sent back to wherever it came from with an explanation of what was missing.

The number of claims received each day by an MCO is very high, running approximately one claim per member per month (and up to three times that rate for

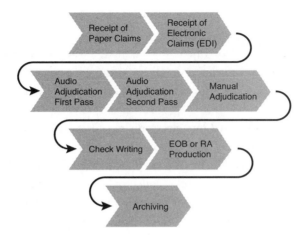

FIGURE 5–4 Claims Capability Operational Functions

Source: Reprinted from D. L. Fowler and E. Pascuzzi, "Claims Administration," in *Essentials of Managed Health Care*, 5th edition, ed. P. R. Kongstvedt (Sudbury, MA: Jones & Bartlett Publishers, 2007), 392.

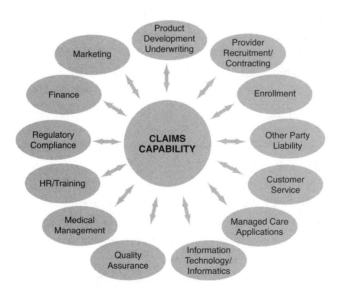

FIGURE 5–5 Claims Capability Relationships within the Managed Care Organization

Source: Reprinted from D. L. Fowler and E. Pascuzzi, "Claims Administration," in *Essentials of Managed Health Care*, 5th edition, ed. P.R. Kongstvedt (Sudbury, MA: Jones & Bartlett Publishers, 2007), 399.

Medicare members).* Even for a medium-sized MCO, it is easy for a claim to get lost in the sheer crush of volume.

Therefore, the claims department, in conjunction with the mailroom, must ensure that all claims are accounted for, either manually or on an automated basis for electronically received claims. Without logging and entry, claims would be impossible to track.

Paper claims are converted into electronic records, first by scanning them into an image file, and then using optical recognition software. Images of those claims that cannot be quickly and easily converted are marked for manual entry. Even a sample of those that are successfully converted may be manually reviewed for quality purposes. These manual interventions are increasingly being carried out securely at off-site locations to save on the cost of labor; all off-site data entry is done using images and electronic records, never actual paper.

Basic Benefits Administration

After capturing the claim, the claims function routinely determines whether the member actually had coverage at the time the claim was incurred, the extent of coverage (i.e., what health services are covered by the MCO), and under what circumstances a benefit does or does not apply.

To illustrate how this works at a high level, a simplified benefits administration scenario for a moderately complex product follows. Most claims are for more straightforward types of plans, such as an HMO or a PPO, but using a moderately complex example illustrates several steps that might or might not occur in different types of plans.

Suppose an employer has purchased a point-of-service (POS; see Chapter 2) benefits package that provides for a $20 copay with no deductible for visits to a primary care physician (PCP), a $35 copay with no deductible for specialist visits authorized by the PCP, and a 30 percent coinsurance requirement with a $500 deductible for services not authorized by the PCP. For purposes if this illustration, we will look at what happens when a claim from a physician comes in for a member enrolled in that employer's POS plan.

Note that in most modern MCOs, all these activities are automated and usually do not require manual intervention. The example will illustrate how the sys-

---

* Data courtesy of Accenture from their proprietary 2007 Healthcare Payer High Performing Metrics Study.

tem works, but at any point, an error or data problem could "kick" the claim out for manual review and processing.

Determining Level of Coverage

When a claim first comes in and after it has been captured, the claims system first checks the enrollment system (see preceding section), which is almost always separate from the claims system, even when both functions are provided by a single IT vendor (i.e., software company). If the membership system indicates that the member was indeed covered, then the claim proceeds to processing. If the member did not have coverage, the claim is immediately denied, and the member and physician are notified and provided an explanation. It should be noted that benefits plans frequently change from year to year (e.g., an increase in the copayment), so a claim for a service provided under an earlier benefits plan may be received after a new benefits plan has been put in place, so the claims system must also use the enrollment system to adjudicate the claim under the appropriate benefits plan.

Assuming that the member is indeed covered, the claims system is then responsible for determining what to pay, if anything. As noted in Chapter 3, the same physician may be considered a PCP for one panel of members and a specialty physician for members not enrolled with that physician for primary care. Thus, the claims department must first determine if the service was provided by the submitting physician as a PCP or a specialty physician (based on whether recipient is a member of the physician's primary care panel). If the claim is considered a specialty care claim, the claims department must find out whether the member's PCP authorized the service.

If the service was not authorized, the claims department must determine whether the member has already met his or her deductible (i.e., paid $500 out-of-pocket for other services before this claim was generated). If the deductible has not been met, the claims department applies some of the claim or the entire claim against the deductible, depending on the amount of the claim and the amount of previous claims. For example, if the claim was for $100 and no previous claims had been filed, the $100 goes against the $500 deductible, leaving $400 for the member to pay out-of-pocket before coverage begins. Another example might be that the member has already satisfied $450 of the deductible, so $50 of the claim goes to fully meeting the deductible, then 70 percent of the remaining $50, which equals $35, is paid by the MCO; the member is then responsible for $65 ($50 plus $15).

Pricing Claims Payment

As noted earlier, the claims department must determine the appropriate amount to pay for each submitted claim (or apply against the deductible). Chapter 3 discussed how each MCO has a fee schedule for calculating the proper reimbursement for a procedure or office visit. If a participating provider submits a claim in excess of the maximum allowed in the fee schedule, the provider agrees (through his or her contract with the MCO) to not collect the difference between the claim and the maximum from either the MCO or the member. In some MCOs, however, the fee schedules for different plans differ from each other. For example, the fee schedule for the HMO may be higher or lower than the fee schedule for the PPO. The claims department must determine which schedule is in effect for each claim.

For purposes of calculating how much to apply against a deductible or against coinsurance, only the amount in the fee schedule is used, not what the provider might have billed. For example, if the provider bills $100 but the maximum fee allowed is $50, then only $50 would be applied against the deductible or coinsurance, and the provider could only collect whatever that amount is.

In the case of a claim from a nonparticipating provider (i.e., a provider that does not have a contract with the MCO), the claims department must still apply a maximum allowable fee to determine how much it will reimburse the member (assuming any coverage at all), but the provider is free to bill the member the difference between that fee and the provider's charge.

Application of Medical Policies

In addition to basic benefits administration, the MCO must apply its policies regarding routine medical care and exceptions. Most routine medical policies are fully integrated into the basic claims adjudication system and are applied on an automated basis at the time that the claim is actually adjudicated. Medical policies for exceptions, however, are always done manually by clinically trained personnel.

Routine Medical Policies

Routine medical policies are rules for using clinical information to make commonplace claims payment decisions. For example, one common medical policy is to pay an assistant surgeon no more than 50 percent of the fee that the primary surgeon receives. Another common policy is to pay only for one abdominal procedure even if a surgeon bills for multiple procedures. For example, if the surgeon bills for both a hysterectomy (removal of the uterus) and a laparotomy (incision through the abdominal wall), the MCO would consider the two procedures to make up a single operation and only pay for that.

The other form of medical policy is really a determination of whether a medical procedure or service is even covered at all. The most common examples are cosmetic surgery, or procedures for which there is no clinical evidence that there is any benefit. Another common example would be that once an inexpensive generic alternative becomes available for a particular drug, an MCO might no longer pay for the brand name; related to this, if a drug goes from being prescription only to becoming available over the counter, it will not be covered at all.

A somewhat more complex type of routine medical policy is the determination of under what clinical circumstances a medical service will be covered, and when will it not. For example, surgery for obesity, called bariatric surgery, may only be covered after evidence of failure of other approaches to weight loss have been documented, and even then, coverage may only be allowed if the member goes to a bariatric surgery center under contract with the MCO (i.e., for this procedure, there may be no out-of-network coverage at all). For this to be automated, the medical management system must create a special authorization, having captured and reviewed appropriate data and then having determined that such surgery met the criteria for coverage. In many cases, medical review is indeed manual, even when processing the claim is automated.

Medical Policies for Exceptions

Some medical policies pertain to coverage for services that are not necessarily covered in the benefits plan. Some exceptions routinely are made; for example, it is rare for MCOs to pay for cosmetic surgery, but they will pay for reconstructive surgery following trauma. Medical policies for exceptions also come into play when a claim arrives for a service that does not match up to the diagnosis that the service is supposed to be for. This usually requires additional information from the provider to resolve the "diagnosis-procedure" mismatch.

More difficult is the issue of experimental or investigational treatments. Until recently, no health plans paid for such treatments, but many lawsuits have compelled MCOs to pay for them even in the absence of clinical data supporting their use. The merits of such lawsuits are, for our purposes, beside the point, and strong arguments in support of any position on this issue can be constructed. What is to the point is that many state legislatures, as well as the federal government, have begun to apply a standard that requires coverage for investigational treatments undertaken as part of approved clinical research. When the demand for an experimental treatment does not take place in the context of an approved investigational program, all the emotionally painful and scientifically difficult issues remain. In any case, the claims department's role is to pend the claim (hold it for further review) until the MCO's medical management function is able to make a determination regarding coverage.

Management of Pended or Appealed Claims and Adjustments

When a claim is pended, the claims department must have a system in place to make sure that the claim does not wind up in limbo. The department needs to track each pended claim and make sure that action ultimately is taken. Reasons that a claim might be pended include the need to allow the medical department to review the claim for medical necessity, confirm that the member was eligible for services when it is not clear, or determine whether another party (e.g., another health insurance company) is primarily responsible for paying the claim.

Other Party Liability

Other party liability (OPL) means that more than one party is potentially liable to pay for a medical service. In the most common case, an individual is covered by two or more health policies, as happens when both members of a married couple are working and have employment-related health benefits. Unless each spouse took single coverage (i.e., coverage for the individual, not the entire family), two policies will be in force, and any children in the family will be covered under two different benefits plans. OPL can also occur in cases in which auto insurance comes into play (because the medical costs are associated with an auto accident) or if a government agency is the primary insurer.

MCOs, health insurers, and other types of insurers follow a complex set of rules in determining which one of several policies has primary payment responsibility and which policies are secondary. Benefits from two policies may also be available under certain circumstances. The same goes for benefits resulting from coverage through some type of government agency or department, and from private insurance coverage. In all cases, a special function of the claims department is to deal with primary liability issues so that the MCO pays what it is supposed to but does not pay when another organization is obligated instead.

Management of Claims Inventory

If all the data have been received in a timely fashion and are accurate, the claim may be processed quickly and correctly, often in less than a week. If, however, the member's enrollment file is not up to date (e.g., the member recently switched to a new PCP but the change was not entered into the system), the claim arrived before the authorization did (e.g., the claim was sent electronically but the mailed authorization arrived 3 days later), or there were data entry errors on the claim, the claim may be processed incorrectly. Therefore, the claims department must have processes in place to prevent these types of common errors from occurring.

If the claims department processes claims with undue delay, several problems may arise. First, of course, providers and members will become unhappy. They have a right to expect their claims to be processed quickly and efficiently. Further, if a backlog builds, providers are likely to send in duplicate claims in the belief (sometimes correct) that the original claims were lost. Duplicate claims add to the volume of claims that the MCO must deal with, and they increase the chance that an error will occur. For example, the MCO might wind up paying the second claim as well as the original, and would then be faced with the task of collecting the overpayment from the provider who received it.

Many states, as well as large employers, have standards for how quickly a "clean claim" must be paid (a clean claim is a claim for which reasons to delay payment are absent). A clean claim usually must be paid in under 15 days, but sometimes only 7 days are allowed. Most MCO contracts with providers allow up to 30 days for payment of a clean claim. Claims that would be considered not clean include duplicate claims, claims with coding errors, claims with other party liability, and claims for nonauthorized services.

Payment and Evidence of Benefit Statements

Once a claim has been approved and finalized, it is routed to the accounts payable function in the system. How the claim is paid depends on who is receiving the money and what, if any, agreements are in place. It is common for hospitals to be paid using electronic funds transfer (EFT), and physicians are increasingly signing up for this as well. The advantages are obvious—payment is received faster, and there is less chance of a check getting lost in the mail or misplaced after it is received. Of course, the provider has to work with the MCO to set up EFT, but that is easily done.

The other form of payment is a paper check, which is mailed. If the provider participates in the MCO's network, the check is mailed directly to the provider. If the provider does not participate (i.e., does not have a contract with the MCO), several options exist. Some providers send in the claim to the MCO as a courtesy to their patient, after asking the patient to sign a form that assigns benefits. Assignment of benefits refers to an agreement between the provider and the patient to ask the MCO to send the check directly to the provider rather than to the subscriber. Some service plans, such as Blue Cross Blue Shield plans, may refuse to assign benefits to a nonparticipating provider, because direct payment is one of the primary benefits of participation. If the member does not assign benefits or if the member paid the provider directly and is seeking reimbursement, the MCO sends the check directly to the subscriber.

Along with either the check or a notification of payment if EFT was used, the MCO also issues an evidence of benefits (EOB) statement. These statements inform the subscriber as to exactly what was paid and what was not, what adjustments were made and why, and how much (if anything) the subscriber may need to pay. The EOB also informs the subscriber of the various ways that he or she can dispute or appeal a payment decision (the appeals process is discussed in the next section). For Medicare, a standardized version is used by all MCOs that provide services to Medicare beneficiaries. Otherwise, an MCO is free to design the EOB any way it wants, as long as it contains certain required information.

Archiving

The final step in the process is storing all the information used to adjudicate the claim, as well as information about how it was finalized. These records are extremely important, especially in cases of appeals and grievances or in the event of a lawsuit. They are also extremely sensitive, so great care is taken to protect privacy. Archival is electronic these days, with even the paper stored to electronic images. Any paper received by the MCO is also stored. Archival is done both on-site at the MCO for ease of retrieval, and off-site at a secure location so that in the event of a disaster, the MCO can still recover necessary information.

Productivity and Quality Management

Productivity and quality management consists of activities intended to ensure that mistakes made in processing claims are kept to a minimum and that the claims department operates as efficiently as possible. Claims department managers measure how many claims a processor handles per day, the accuracy (or conversely, the error rate) of the claims that are processed, the types of problems that occur with high frequency so that the cause of the problem may be addressed, and so forth. Managers of the claims department also look for ways to improve efficiency, such as using electronic imaging to capture paper documents, using electronic access to medical policy documentation, and other labor-saving approaches. The greater the automation of the claims process, the higher the quality and efficiency of the process.

THE BANKING FUNCTION*

With the advent of CDHPs, a new need for managing the banking function has arisen. As described in Chapter 2, CDHPs use some sort of savings option that accumulates pretax dollars for use in paying for at least some of the health care that is received while the member is still subject to the high deductible. The typical CDHP is a high-deductible group benefits plan with a pretax health reimbursement account (HRA), whereas an individual HDHP may or may not have an associated pretax health savings account (HSA). Unused funds in an HRA or HSA may roll over for use in future years, though certain rules and limitations apply.

A third type of pretax savings account is called a flexible spending account (FSA), which may be used for health care expenses and/or child care expenses. FSAs are regulated differently than health insurance is, and they are independent of an HRA or an HSA. Only a small amount of any unused FSA funds may roll over to the next year.

Although it is common for a bank or financial services company of some sort to manage the HRA, HSA, or FSA, some MCOs are now offering these banking services directly (this is now legal with the repeal some years ago of a depression-era law that prohibited insurance companies from running banks and vice versa). Even if an MCO does not offer banking services themselves, they still may team up with a bank to do so. In both cases, the MCO offers to automatically deduct the required funds from the HRA or HSA either to pay the provider or to send a check to the subscriber. Without such an arrangement, the subscriber must submit evidence of payment to the bank to receive a check. Finally, not all expenses are considered eligible for reimbursement by an HRA, HSA, or FSA, and the banking function must verify that they meet certain criteria.

MEMBER SERVICES

The member services department acts as the interface between members and the MCO. In other words, when an individual member has a problem or needs assistance, it is member services that provides the necessary assistance. Member services is responsible for many functions, but only the most important are discussed here (Exhibit 5–2). Interactions between members and member services may occur on the

---

* Get set for an especially heavy dose of acronyms.

EXHIBIT 5-2

Responsibilities of Member Services

Provide general information to members.

Provide routine communication to certain members.

Address member problems, complaints, appeals, and grievances.

Provide proactive outreach to members.

Perform continual surveillance and analysis of member satisfaction.

telephone, via secure e-mail, by using secure live Web-enabled chat, by U.S. mail (or any other document delivery service), or face to face in a customer service center.

Provision of General Information

An MCO is in constant need of communicating with its members. The communication process begins before enrollment, when the MCO must provide information to prospective enrollees so they can make informed decisions, such as whether to join the plan and what PCP to select. It then continues throughout the enrollee's membership in the MCO and even beyond.

The MCO must routinely provide updated lists of participating providers, changes in hours of operations, changes in medical policies, and the like. It should also regularly offer educational information, such as health tips, immunization schedules, and smoking cessation and other forms of preventive medical education.

Routine Communication

Besides general information provided to all members, an MCO also needs to communicate specific information to certain members. Examples include changes in the health benefits plan of a particular employer or changes in the drug formulary that will change coverage levels for certain drugs. In these cases, the member services department communicates the necessary information to any members who are affected by the change.

Some routine communications are required by law or regulation. For example, under the Consolidated Omnibus Reconciliation Act (COBRA), an MCO must notify members leaving the health plan of their rights regarding continuation of coverage as discussed in Chapter 7. It must also notify members about privacy and confidentiality (also discussed in Chapter 7), reimbursement policies, and appeal and grievance rights, as discussed next.

Addressing Member Problems, Complaints, Appeals, and Grievances

Working with members to manage problems, complaints, appeals, and grievances is perhaps the most important function performed by member services. MCOs are required to address member problems and other issues under state and federal laws and regulations, although the specifics of the requirements vary from state to state. For members covered under self-funded plans, the federal Employee Retirement Income Security Act (ERISA) prevails. For members covered under fully insured policies, both ERISA and state laws apply. This very important topic is also discussed further in Chapter 7.

Member problems range from something as simple as an incorrect identification card to something as complex as a mishandled claim for medical expenses. MCOs have a special interest in helping members select physicians in an HMO or a POS plan and straightening out problems with authorization and other unique aspects of managed care.

Members have the right to file a formal complaint. Although a member may bring a complaint based on his or her first contact with the MCO (e.g., a complaint about rude or unprofessional behavior by a provider), most complaints stem from problems that are not resolved to the members' satisfaction. For example, an MCO may deny a medical claim on the grounds that the service in question is not covered, but the member might disagree.

All MCOs have rules and procedures in place for the resolution of complaints. The rules might require timelines for responding to a complaint (e.g., a response must be made within 30 days), require the existence of formal tracking mechanisms, and define who must review particular types of complaints and respond to them (e.g., the medical director might have to review all medically related complaints, whereas an appropriate vice president might have to review all complaints about member services). The entire review process and all communications with the member are carefully documented.

An appeal is a formal request for review of a decision regarding coverage for specified medical costs or procedures. In most states, an appeal of a coverage decision requires an external review of the decision. In an external review, physicians who are not employed by the MCO and are otherwise independent of it review the case and reach a determination. Again, detailed rules apply to an external review, and there is a timeline for the entire process. In some cases, a special "expedited review" is required, such as when the medical procedure is urgent (e.g., an experimental transplant). The conclusion reached by the review panel is usually binding on the MCO. Under ERISA, members (regardless of whether they are in an insured or a self-funded plan) also have appeal rights to have their case reviewed by a neutral third party, including an expedited appeal, but whether a physician must be involved or the review done by an external reviewer is less clear.

A grievance is a special type of formal complaint and requires a formal response by the MCO. The response must follow specific guidelines, although these tend to differ from state to state. Federal programs such as Medicare also have formal grievance procedures.

Grievances, as compared with other types of complaints, are especially likely to involve an external agency, usually a government one. A federal agency may be drawn in if the grievance is brought by an enrollee in Medicare or the Federal Employees Health Benefits Program, and the relevant state insurance department may be drawn in if the grievance is brought by an enrollee in a commercial insurance plan or HMO. The grievance procedures of a health plan self-funded by the employer must meet requirements mandated by ERISA, but members covered under self-funded plans have less recourse to a government agency for grievances.

Grievance procedures can differ from one type of coverage to another, but in all cases, they include formal hearings and testimony (in the MCO, not a court of law) and have timeline and documentation requirements. If the grievance procedures do not result in an outcome satisfactory to the member, the member may still have recourse to an external agency or to the courts, though there are limitations even there for members in self-funded plans.

Proactive Outreach

If all that a member services department did was handle problems, complaints, appeals, and grievances, it would not be filling its real potential. Proactively reaching out to members can have a powerful impact on member satisfaction and on the operations of the MCO. For instance, a welcoming call to new members can help them understand how the MCO operates, answer any questions they have, and take care of any issues that may have already arisen. Contacting members who have not extensively used the MCO's services is one way to make sure that they are satisfied with their membership.

Surveillance and Analysis of Member Satisfaction

An MCO must continually gauge the level of member satisfaction. Periodic surveys will allow the MCO to discover how members view their health plans and to pick up on trends early on. A survey may contain general questions intended to expose the overall level of satisfaction with the MCO, or it may contain narrow questions targeted at specific issues, such as the adequacy of the provider network. In some cases, formal member satisfaction surveys are compulsory (e.g., Medicare mandates their use), and these surveys are created by a federal agency. Further, to obtain external accreditation (see Chapter 7), an MCO must perform broad member satisfaction surveys and act on the results. In recent years, the federal surveys have also been adopted by accreditation agencies to provide for more consistent information.

FINANCE

The finance department of an MCO is responsible for managing the money. The most important of their many functions are described next, after the following brief account of the financial measures used in MCOs.

Perhaps the most common unit of measure is per member per month (PMPM). To illustrate, suppose the finance department reports that the cost of the drug benefit for a particular health benefits plan is $40 PMPM. That means that on average, the monthly cost for every member with that drug benefits plan is $40. The monthly cost for one particular member might be $800, and it might be zero for another member, but it averages $40.

The other two measures—whole dollars and percent of premium—are even easier to understand. The first, whole dollars, is just what it sounds like—the total amount spent (or, in the case of income, the total amount received in the form of premium payments). The second measure, which is also what it sounds like, is easiest to understand in the context of reporting costs. For example, the cost of hospital care may represent 35 percent of each premium dollar (i.e., for each dollar of premium collected, $0.35 goes toward paying for hospital care). Whole dollars and percent of premium are usually reported for each month and for the year (or year to date).

The following illustrates various ways of reporting the same results. Assume that the MCO collects, in the form of premium payments, $275 PMPM, spends 35 percent of each dollar received on hospital care, and has 100,000 members covered under the health benefits plan. The amount collected equals $275 PMPM, which is $27,500,000 per month in whole dollars ($275 × 100,000), and

$330,000,000 per year in whole dollars ($27,500,000 × 12). As for hospital costs, they equal 35 percent of the premium collected, or $96.25 PMPM ($275 × 0.35), which is $9,625,000 per month in whole dollars ($27,500,000 × 0.35), and $115,500,000 per year in whole dollars ($330,000,000 × 0.35).

The other commonly used metric is member months, though it's not usually used by itself. The term refers to the number of members covered each month, added together. For example, if 100,000 members were covered in one month, 110,000 members were covered in the second month, and 105,000 members were covered in the third month, total member months for that 3-month period would be 315,000 (100,000 + 110,000 + 105,000). Members are only counted in the member month calculation if they are subject to whatever the finance department is looking at. For example, a member who does not have a drug benefit would not be included if the finance department was calculating costs for pharmacy. Using member months allows the finance department to more easily calculate something on a PMPM basis. For example, if the MCO paid out a total of $15,000,000.00 for prescription drugs in the first quarter of the year, and the first quarter of the year had 315,000 member months (of members with the drug benefit), then the cost of the drug benefit was $47.62 PMPM.

Operational Finance

Operational finance refers to the day-to-day functions of the finance department. The most important of these functions are tracking all money that moves in to and out of the MCO, tracking where it goes, identifying how much goes where, and noting why it does so. Following is a brief review of the major areas managed by the finance department.

Premium Revenue

The first step in the financial process is to receive the premium payments owed. These are actually accounted for by the finance department before the money arrives. The revenue at this point is referred to as accrued revenue or booked revenue; it is referred to as cash revenue after the actual receipt of the money. Why the difference? Because the MCO must know ahead of time how much money it expects to receive and to account for that money properly. Over time, the finance department (along with the billing and enrollment departments) must reconcile the amount of money paid by an employer (or government agency) against the amount the MCO believes it is owed based on the enrolled members. The total amount of premium owed is, of course, equal to the number of enrollees and the premium (i.e., price) of the health benefits plan.

Medical Costs

The next step is to determine where the money is to go. The majority of the money, between 80 and 85 percent in most cases, goes toward medical costs. As described in prior chapters, there are many types of providers and medical services. It is up to the finance department to track how much money goes for each type of service and to each provider. For example, most MCOs usually track how much money is being spent on:

- Primary care vs. specialty care (HMOs only)
- Physician care in total
- Hospital or other inpatient institutional care
- Ambulatory surgery or outpatient procedures
- Behavioral health services
- Diagnostics and ancillary services
- Prescription drugs
- Emergency or urgent care

In reality, well-run MCOs track cost in even more categories—for example, specialty pharmacy, specialized imaging, high-cost ("catastrophic") cases, and the like. The MCO will also usually track medical expenses by major line of business. For example, Medicare is tracked separately from commercial business; small-group business, large-group business, and self-insured business are tracked separately; and so forth.

Note that an MCO must book expenses for medical services well before it receives claims for those services. If the MCO were to book expenses only for claims it has actually received, it would seriously miscalculate what the costs will eventually total. For instance, the costs of medical services are influenced by changes in membership numbers, the health benefits plans in force, and seasonality (medical costs vary depending on the season; for example, little elective surgery is scheduled over Thanksgiving). The finance department must estimate what the costs are going to be and reserve enough money to pay for them.

An MCO puts aside money in a reserve—known as the IBNR (incurred but not reported)—to pay for medical claims that come in over time but about which it does not know any specifics. There are numerous techniques that the finance department, with help from the actuarial and underwriting departments, uses to calculate the IBNR. The point here is that the finance department has the responsibility to ensure that the MCO has put aside sufficient funds to pay for medical expenses.

Administrative Costs

Administrative costs fall into many categories. Many MCOs track a very large number of different categories of administrative costs so as to better manage them. Common categories include at least:

- Marketing and sales
- Member services
- Medical management
- Network management
- Finance
- Actuarial and underwriting
- Legal
- Claims
- Enrollment and billing
- Information systems
- Occupancy (e.g., the cost of the occupying office space, cost to run the mail room, etc.)

The Bottom Line

Finally, the finance function of the MCO must calculate the bottom line, or how much money is left after paying all medical and administrative costs. In almost all cases, MCOs, even nonprofit MCOs, are subject to taxation. Therefore, the cost of taxes must also be taken into account. After that, the profit (in the case of a for-profit MCO) or reserve position (in the case of a nonprofit MCO) is reported.

Treasury

The treasury function within the finance department is responsible for actually managing the cash and investments of the MCO. An MCO must maintain adequate financial reserves to cover the cost of claims, and most states require an MCO to maintain reserves sufficient to cover approximately 2–3 months' worth of claims even if no more money was received by the MCO; the actual reserve requirement is calculated using a complex formula called "risk-based capital," which is beyond the scope of this book. To properly manage those reserves, the MCO rarely uses cash, but instead invests that money in very secure types of investments that can easily be cashed out. Any money in excess of the actual reserve requirement may be used in other types of investments, but MCOs generally avoid investments that have any significant degree of risk. Self-funded employers do not pay premiums to the MCO. When claims are paid for members in self-funded plans, the MCO notifies the employer of the amount. That amount is then transferred electronically to a lock box (not a real lock box, but an electronic one), and the claims are paid using those funds. An MCO is not required to maintain any reserves for self-funded plans because it is not at risk for those expenses; the employer is.

Finally, it is the treasury function that must ensure that there is cash on hand to pay all the expenses of the MCO. These expenses include not only claims but also all the costs to actually run the company, including paying the employees, though most MCOs use an outside company to actually administer payroll.

Budgeting

All organizations require a budget to properly manage operations, and MCOs are no different. What makes budgeting for an MCO unique is the need to create a budget for medical expenses and a separate one for operational expenses. Further, different financial tools and techniques are used to create the two budgets. Budgeting is essential, for it is only through the budget process that the MCO can test assumptions about how much to charge in premium or determine what enhanced systems capabilities the MCO will be able to afford. Operational budgets must actually address two general categories: what must be spent to simply run the MCO, and what can be spent to improve operations (which includes both enhancing services and spending money to improve efficiencies to lower costs).

Reporting

Reporting is discussed apart from budgeting because there are several types of reporting that the finance department must do. It is the finance department that is usually responsible for creating reports for each employer, the U.S. Department of Labor, Medicare, and so forth, and sending them to the appropriate recipients. Some large MCOs use a separate analytics department to create reports as well. An independent form of reporting known as internal audit also frequently resides in the finance department and is responsible for ensuring that all areas of the MCO are both reporting accurate numbers and operating according to the company's policies and guidelines.

Using special forms, the MCO must report financial and utilization results to the state insurance departments of those states in which it does business, although in some cases, a state insurance department will accept the results that have been reported to the insurance department of the state in which the MCO is based. Reporting financial status to the state is not an easy task, at least with regard to insured business, because the MCO must use a type of accounting based on statutory accounting principles (SAP) rather than the type based on generally accepted accounting principles (GAAP); the differences between SAP and GAAP are beyond the scope of this book, however. Each MCO must also produce quarterly and annual reports containing both GAAP and SAP accounting information.

Finally, the finance department is responsible for maintaining the financial records in such a manner as to be considered acceptable to an independent external auditor. For-profit plans must have their annual statements certified by an accredited auditing firm, and under a new federal law, the chief executive officer must attest to the accuracy of the financial statements.

Actuarial Services

The job of the actuarial services department is to estimate future medical expenses. The estimates are influenced by the design of the benefits plan, changes in laws (e.g., the mandating of certain benefits), the configuration of the network (e.g., fee schedules), assumptions about utilization patterns, and so forth. The actuarial services department also examines the IBNR calculations to ensure that an adequate amount of money has been set aside to pay for future medical claims.

Small and midsized MCOs may contract with external actuarial firms rather than hire staff actuaries. Even when an MCO does have staff actuaries, it is standard for outside actuaries to examine the IBNR and claims reserves as part of the annual audit.

Underwriting

Underwriting is related to estimating medical expenses, although it is done by nonactuaries. The two primary activities of the underwriting department are rate development and determining the level of risk of medical costs.

Rate Development

Underwriters are charged with using the cost estimates prepared by the finance and actuarial services departments to calculate the actual premium rates that the

MCO will charge customers. There are many types of rating, each useful in different circumstances. Following is a brief description of the most common.

Standard community rating. In this type of rating, an MCO creates a standard set of rates that it charges everyone regardless of differences in the size or makeup of the employer groups. For example, if the MCO determines that it needs $275 PMPM in revenue for a particular insured product, it creates rates that will yield that amount, and that is what it charges. This does not mean there is a monthly premium rate of $275 for each person, because the revenue requirement was based on a mix of adults and children. The rate charged to a person with only single coverage (i.e., coverage only for herself or himself) is always higher than the PMPM revenue requirement, whereas family rates are usually lower than what they would be if each person were charged $275. The reason is that the medical costs for children are far less than for adults. Standard community rating is mostly used in the small-group market, and in many states, it is the only type of rating allowed in the small-group market.

Adjusted community rating and community rating by class. In adjusted community rating, an MCO calculates a standard community rate and then adjusts it based on a number of variables. The most common factors influencing the adjustment are the anticipated average size of families and the proportion of families versus the proportion of single individuals. If families are small, less revenue is needed for each family, for example; even though children are less expensive than adults, if there are fewer of them, there are simply fewer people being covered. Another factor, although it is less commonly used, is the employer's type of business, because certain types of businesses are considered higher risk than others; for example, commercial fishermen are at greater risk of injury than are accountants. This type of rating may or may not be used in the small-group market, but it is often used in the midsized market when groups are too small to properly experience rate.

Experience rating. This type of rating reflects the actual medical experience of the employer group. If the group has had high medical expenses in the past, it will be charged a higher premium than a group whose medical costs have been low. Experience rating depends on the ability to differentiate between trends and just plain bad luck. For example, a group may have high expenses one year because of a single terrible auto accident (such cases are sometimes referred to as "shock claims"). Another group's high expenses, on the other hand, may be due to the fact that all the employees and their families smoke asbestos while riding motorcycles under the influence of alcohol. The first group's history of high expenses was owing to bad luck and does not indicate that its expenses will remain high, whereas the high expenses of the second group are guaranteed to continue. Thus, experience rating is used only for groups with enough enrollees to allow the MCO to determine whether their history of medical costs reflects actual trends.

Rating for self-insured employers. Even the account of a self-insured employer needs to have "rates" calculated so that the employer knows the likely future cost of employee health benefits, and the employees can be charged for whatever portion is their responsibility. Although these are not true premium rates, they are often referred to as a "premium equivalent" because they perform much the same function.

Determining the Level of Risk

The other major activity of the underwriting department is to determine the level of risk of medical costs. Actuaries determine the overall risk of medical costs, but it is up to the underwriters to apply those principles to new employer groups or individuals applying for health insurance coverage. The underwriters take many factors into account, including past medical claims history, current medical conditions, and so forth. In some cases, such as mandated open enrollment periods or in states that require MCOs to issue coverage to small groups regardless of their past history of costs, the underwriting department has little effect. Otherwise, when an employer seeks coverage from the MCO, the department analyzes the relevant factors and determines whether to offer coverage, what products to offer, and what rates to charge for those products.

INFORMATION TECHNOLOGY

An MCO's IT system comprises the computer hardware and software and the telecommunications technologies that it uses to store and transmit information. The overall information system will typically include a mainframe system to handle day-to-day operations, an internal network to allow electronic communication within the MCO, Internet or e-commerce capabilities for communication with the outside world, and telephone systems. It will also likely include private communications systems for business-to-business electronic interchange, data storage and analysis systems, and so forth.

The information system constitutes the backbone of the MCO's operations. All the activities described in this chapter and others depend on computer hardware and software, and if the information system is not working efficiently and properly, the MCO's ability to manage its finances, maintain membership data, process claims, and manage medical cases will be diminished. Therefore, the information system must be updated continually, and the various hardware and software problems that plague every MCO must be addressed promptly.

The MCO's ability to conduct business with other parties, such as providers and employers, also depends on its information system. Great quantities of paper are still used in the transaction of business, but paper is rapidly being replaced by electronic forms of information storage and transmission. Under HIPAA, the numerous conflicting standards for electronic transactions were made uniform, which has led to increasing adoption of electronic transactions as the norm. HIPAA, including the mandated transactions and code sets, are discussed in Chapter 7.

Finally, most MCOs have a department dedicated to using data for analytic purposes. This function, often referred to as informatics, may be very focused in particular areas, such as medical costs, or it may be more generalized, such as creating ever more useful operational reports for managers. Regardless, an informatics capability is becoming increasingly important for MCOs to succeed in today's market.

CONCLUSION

Although 80–85 percent of each dollar of premium is spent on clinical services, administrative activities make up most of what an MCO does from day to day. The MCO's normal functions include enrolling members, billing for and receiving premium payments, processing authorizations and other aspects of medical management, and paying claims. In addition, the MCO must ensure that it has the means to help members resolve problems and manage complaints, appeals, and grievances. Finally, it must have the appropriate staff, as well as the appropriate information technologies, for managing its finances. Because of the complexity of its normal operations, the administrative challenges facing the typical MCO would be hard to overestimate.

Medicare and Medicaid

Managed care organizations (MCOs) offer services to a variety of market segments. For most MCOs, the most important segment is the commercial market, consisting of employers that offer health insurance or managed care coverage to their employees. A related segment is made up of individual purchasers of coverage, but individual coverage and group coverage operate in much the same way (see Chapter 5 for an account of the differences). The focus of this chapter is on two "noncommercial" market segments—Medicare and Medicaid. As the commercial market has become more and more competitive, most MCOs have turned increasingly to the noncommercial market for growth. Furthermore, there are now many local MCOs and national companies that focus solely on these segments, and on Medicaid in particular.

As an aside, the reader will note that these two programs share a trait found in many government programs: the extensive use of acronyms (i.e., using initials as shorthand). Managed care uses acronyms itself—MCO is one example—but their use in Medicare and Medicaid far exceeds anything found in the commercial sector. In fact, it is the author's opinion that only the military uses more acronyms than do governmental health programs. To quote Carlos Zarabozo (see Note 3, p. 162): "TGIF—The Government is Frightening, unless you know your acronyms." To assist the reader, only a small number of the more commonly used acronyms will be used in this chapter.

MEDICARE

Medicare, which began in 1965, is the most important health care entitlement program in the nation. It provides health care benefits for the elderly, for persons with end-stage renal disease (i.e., kidney failure), and for some disabled persons. The traditional Medicare program consists of Part A (benefits for hospital services) and Part B (benefits for medical services), which has operated as a fee-for-service program. Typically, the federal government contracts with fiscal intermediaries (e.g., nongovernment organizations such as Blue Cross and Blue Shield plans) to process Medicare claims; in other words, providers bill the fiscal intermediaries for services received by Medicare beneficiaries, and the intermediaries process the claims on behalf of Medicare. Traditional Medicare has a rigid schedule of maximum fees based on the resource-based relative value scale for professionals and a variety of payment mechanisms for hospitals, nursing homes, ambulatory surgical centers, and so forth; these reimbursement methodologies are discussed in Chapter 3.

Beginning in 1985, Medicare allowed MCOs to offer services under Medicare Part C. Medicare beneficiaries were able to enroll in health maintenance organizations (HMOs) and be treated like commercial members, although the HMOs were subject to special rules regarding sales and marketing, reporting, and reimbursement. Later, the Balanced Budget Act of 1997 (BBA) expanded the benefits options and the plans available under Medicare to include Medicare HMOs, Medicare preferred provider organizations (PPOs), Medicare point-of-service plans (POS), a new type of Medicare plan called private fee-for-service (PFFS), provider-sponsored organizations (PSOs), and a demonstration program for medical savings accounts (MSAs), all of which are described later in this chapter. These various nontraditional options were in a program then called Medicare+Choice.

In 2003, the Medicare Prescription Drug Improvement and Modernization Act was passed by Congress and signed into law. This act, which came to be known as the Medicare Modernization Act (MMA), created a new benefit, Medicare Part D, that added drug coverage as a Medicare benefit nearly 40 years after the beginning of Medicare. Under the MMA, Part C, the old Medicare+Choice program, became the Medicare Advantage (MA) program.

To briefly summarize what the MMA did with respect to health plans, it provided more money for health plans in a variety of ways. In addition, the MMA introduced a new approach to plan contracting: the regional plan option. The Centers for Medicare and Medicaid Services (CMS), that part of the federal Department of Health and Human Services (DHHS) that oversees Medicare, divided the United States into 26 regions within which organizations agreeing to function as PPOs that serve an entire region would offer those PPO plans to Medicare beneficiaries. Existing Medicare+Choice plans of all types became known as MA-local plans to distinguish them from the new regional PPOs. In addition to requiring that regional plans be set up as PPOs offered in every county of a region, payment rules and certain contracting provisions are different for regional plans. To encourage the growth of regional PPOs, CMS did not allow any new local plans to start up for two years, but in 2008, that restriction was removed.

The MMA also created a new type of MA plan—the Special Needs Plan (SNP). An SNP may exclusively enroll, or enroll a disproportionate percentage of, special needs Medicare beneficiaries. Individuals with special needs include beneficiaries entitled to both Medicare and Medicaid ("dual eligibles" or "duals"), institutionalized beneficiaries, and individuals with severe or disabling chronic conditions. SNPs are also discussed later in this chapter in the section on Medicaid.

The Medicare Part D Drug Benefit in Medicare Advantage

All MA organizations other than PFFS plans and MSA plans (both described later in this chapter) are required to offer a plan with Medicare Part D drug coverage throughout their service area. Organizations are free to offer plans that do not include drug coverage (for beneficiaries who elect to decline drug coverage). PFFS plans can include Part D drug coverage, but MSA plans are not permitted to include Part D coverage as part of the plan.

The MMA added drug coverage as a benefit to be administered by private entities, either "stand-alone" prescription drug plans (PDPs) or Medicare Advantage Prescription Drug (MA-PD) plans.[1] The benefit is voluntary for regular Medicare beneficiaries, but dual eligibles (having both Medicare and Medicaid) are automatically in the program. It is primarily paid for by federal subsidies, with a portion of the voluntary benefit paid by beneficiaries in the form of premiums and cost sharing, and a portion financed by plans that are partly at risk for the provision of the benefit. Access standards apply to ensure that beneficiaries have convenient access to pharmacies.

The basic Part D benefit (referred to as the "defined standard" benefit) is complicated and is characterized by a "donut hole," which refers to a coverage gap that appears at a certain point and during which an enrollee who has no low-income subsidy is responsible for 100 percent of the cost of drugs (though they can still purchase their medicines at the discounted rate that his or her plan offers).

The specific minimum Part D benefit is as follows. After a small deductible ($265 in 2007[2]), the beneficiary then pays 25 percent of the cost of a covered Part D prescription drug up to an initial coverage limit ($2,400 in 2007). On reaching that point—the donut hole—the beneficiary pays 100 percent of the cost of drugs (up to $3,051 in 2007) until total expenditures reach $5,451 (representing $3,850 in "true out of pocket costs" for the beneficiary in 2007). At that point, catastrophic coverage begins. Under the standard benefit, catastrophic coverage has the beneficiary paying only 5 percent coinsurance (unless the person is a low-income beneficiary entitled to a subsidy that would pick up even the coinsurance).

In reality, MA-PDs and PDPs usually offer benefits that are a bit easier to understand, using fixed-dollar-amount copayments rather than percentage coinsurance. These plans also use formularies, providing for higher levels of coverage for less expensive drugs such as generics. Some plans even offer coverage of certain generic drugs during the donut hole portion of the benefit. No plan may offer less coverage than the standard benefit, however.

The bidding process for how CMS determines its portion of the costs is highly complicated and well beyond the scope of this book, but part of the process involves setting a target for the overall cost for drugs provided to enrollees, adjusted

---

[1] Residents of long-term care (LTC) facilities obtain drug benefits from the pharmacy selected by the facility. There is a special enrollment period for people who enter, reside in, or leave a LTC facility.

[2] The specific dollar amounts of the deductible, initial coverage limits, and catastrophic threshold change from year to year based on certain inflation indexes.

for how sick they are. Through 2011, the federal government shares both the risk and reward with MA-PDs and PDPs if costs either significantly exceed or fall below that target, though the amount of risk and reward sharing gets lower each year. After 2011, there is likely to remain some amount of risk and reward sharing, but the amount will be determined at a future date. Finally, the federal government provides subsidies for providing the benefit to low-income individuals.

Medicare Advantage Managed Care Plans

The first requirement for any organization to become an MA plan is to be licensed in the state in which it operates. For regional plans, it must be licensed in at least one state in the region. There are some exceptions, but this is not common. There are a variety of MA plan types, but only a designated regional PPO is considered a regional plan, and all other types of plans are considered "local." MA plans are also categorized as either coordinated care plans (including HMOs, PPOs, PSOs, and POS plans, all described more fully in Chapter 2) or non–coordinated care plans (PFFS plans and MSA plans). The main difference is that coordinated care plans can require a Medicare member to use a contracted provider for all but emergency services. MA local plans may also offer an MA service area that is smaller than the service area of the commercial health plans, as long as the MA service area does not skip over a county. Finally, there are special provisions under the MMA for employer-sponsored MA plans, but those too are beyond the scope of this book.

Traditional Medicare HMOs

Traditional Medicare HMOs are similar to the Medicare managed care plans that existed even prior to the BBA. They are licensed by the state (see Chapter 7 for a discussion of state licensure) or at least are subject to oversight by the state (e.g., a Medicaid-only HMO that is not licensed as a commercial HMO but still meets state oversight requirements). In essence, CMS has delegated the oversight of commercial and Medicaid HMOs to the states and accepts state certification as sufficient evidence that an HMO is meeting financial and market conduct standards.

In addition to the relevant state requirements, MA HMOs face additional federal requirements. As one example, an MCO must have at least 5,000 members (or 1,500 members if operating in a rural area) to secure an MA contract, though that can be waived for the first three years of a start-up plan. Other federal requirements are discussed toward the end of the chapter.

Provider-Sponsored Organizations

PSOs, which were enabled under the BBA, are similar to HMOs except that they are owned and operated by the providers themselves. A PSO is an organization in which most services are provided by the sponsoring providers (i.e., the providers that have majority ownership or control of the organization) or affiliated providers (i.e., providers at direct or indirect financial risk for the organization). In particular, in an urban area, 70 percent of health care services (as measured by expenditures) must be provided directly by the sponsoring providers or by affiliated providers (the required proportion is only 60 percent in a rural area).

PSOs were created under the BBA and pertain solely to Medicare Advantage (formerly Medicare+Choice). They may be licensed by the state, in which case they are functionally similar to HMOs, though PSOs may not be required to meet the same solvency standards as state-licensed HMOs. Whereas both HMOs and PSOs must maintain defined levels of liquidity (i.e., cash or cash-equivalent funds) and defined levels of reserves (i.e., money set aside for financially difficult times), the levels required of an HMO are higher than for a PSO. The thinking behind not requiring PSOs to maintain the higher levels is that the providers in a PSO are themselves at risk for services and do not need to worry as much about paying for services to others.

When the BBA was passed, providers greeted the opportunity to create PSOs with enthusiasm. Unfortunately, relatively few PSOs ever got off the ground, and most of those that did lost significant amounts of money. Most of the PSOs created as part of an initial demonstration project went out of existence, and new applicants for PSO status did not finalize the process and become operational. Although PSO status remains an option under the MMA, few PSOs remain in operation. Whether they will ever make a comeback is hard to determine.

Preferred Provider Organizations

MA-local PPOs must be licensed as a risk-bearing entity by the state, whereas regional PPOs can be licensed in only one state within a multistate region. Regional PPOs also differ from MA-local PPOs in how they must administer benefits; regional PPOs are required to have only one deductible that applies to hospital and physician services combined, rather than separately, as in traditional Medicare. In reality, some MA-local PPOs administer the benefit in this way as well.

Although regional PPOs are required to have a network of providers, the access standard can be met by paying for nonnetwork services at Medicare fee-for-service rates. There is also a provision in which Medicare will make payments to an "essential provider," defined as a hospital that is necessary to include in the network but that, after a good faith effort on the part of the plan, does not agree to a contract with payment at Medicare rates.

Point-of-Service Plans

Under MA, MA-HMOs may offer a POS benefit to their Medicare enrollees. In general, a POS benefit allows an enrollee to receive services delivered by out-of-network providers, but the services, although still covered, are subject to a higher deductible and coinsurance. The regulations provide great latitude in the design of the benefit, how it is financed (e.g., it could be offered as an additional benefit funded by Medicare capitation payments), the charges to enrollees, and the extent of its availability (e.g., it could be restricted to retirees of an employer group). However, organizations offering a POS option are subject to additional monitoring by CMS to ensure continued compliance with standards pertaining to financial solvency, availability and accessibility of care, quality assurance, member appeals, and marketing.

Private Fee-for-Service Plans

A PFFS plan is a private health insurance plan that reimburses providers on a fee-for-service basis and does not limit enrollees to the use of network providers. As an enrollee of an MA PFFS plan, a Medicare beneficiary may use any Medicare-participating provider who agrees to provide services to the beneficiary, and the organization sponsoring the PFFS plan (e.g., a private insurer) will pay for covered services in a manner similar to a traditional indemnity plan operating in the private marketplace. A PFFS plan may not pay its providers other than on a fee-for-service basis and may not place providers at financial risk for the utilization of services.

PFFS plans are rather elaborate. To illustrate this, a basic description of a PFFS plan follows:

> The PFFS plan may have a network of providers who agree to the terms of the plan, but the law also provides for "deemed" participating providers. A provider is deemed to be a participating provider if he or she (or the entity) is aware of the beneficiary's enrollment in the PFFS plan and the provider is aware of, or has been given a reasonable opportunity to be made aware of, the terms and conditions of payment under the plan "in a manner reasonably designed to effect informed agreement" to participate, as stated in the regulations. A non-contracting provider may only receive, in total payments (from the PFFS plan and from enrollee cost sharing), an amount equal to what would have been paid in total under traditional Medicare. Contracting and deemed providers may also receive additional

payments from the enrollee ("balance billing") up to 15 percent of the PFFS plan payment amount. The PFFS organization is charged with ensuring that providers adhere to the limits on permissible balance billed amounts; failure to monitor adherence to the requirement can result in CMS's decision not to renew the organization's contract. Enrollees may incur additional liability if the PFFS retrospectively denies coverage (as not Medicare-covered or for non-Medicare-covered benefits not covered under the plan).[3]

Medical Savings Accounts

MSAs authorized under the BBA were a demonstration only, and in fact, few if any were ever even sold. The MMA continued to authorize MSAs, including a new Medicare MSA demonstration program, but participation remains low. MSAs generally are similar to the health savings accounts (HSAs) described in Chapter 2 (in fact, HSAs were created under the MMA, though not for Medicare), in that MSAs are pre-tax funds used to pay for some of the costs incurred before a high-deductible insurance plan begins to provide coverage.

Reimbursement of Medicare Advantage Plans

CMS's method of reimbursing MA plans is complicated, although, as noted in Chapter 5, the pricing and premium payment methods used by commercial products are complicated as well. Payment to plans is based on payment rates established by law and a comparison of these payment rates to plan bids under what is referred to as a competitive bidding system. The bid of a local MA plan for coverage of Medicare A and B services is compared with a benchmark to determine whether there is a premium for Medicare-covered services and to determine the level of "savings" a plan projects if the plan believes that it can provide the Medicare package for less than the benchmark. A plan's bid is affected by whether it thinks it will enroll a population that is either sicker or healthier than average, and CMS adjusts how much it pays the plan based on how sick or healthy an enrolled population is. If the bid is higher than the benchmark, the plan can charge a premium; if it is lower, the plan can provide more services or a reduced premium for Parts B and D. Premiums and benefits under Part D are otherwise addressed

---

[3] Quoted from C. Zarabozo and S. Lindenberg, "Health Plans and Medicare," *The Essentials of Managed Health Care Handbook,* 5th edition, ed. P. R. Kongstvedt (Sudbury, MA: Jones & Bartlett Publishers, 2007), 592.

separately from the basic MA premiums and benefits. Finally, there are some adjustments based on the geography of where enrollment occurs.

An important change in payment policy addresses the issue of "selection bias" among Medicare risk plans (selection bias refers to a plan enrolling members who are healthier or sicker than average). Previously, the payment adjustment factors were limited to demographic factors such as age and sex. CMS payments to health plans are now adjusted at the individual member level by demographic factors *and* health status factors, based on diagnostic information submitted by MA plans. The diagnostic information for the adjustments is based on a minimum data set submitted by health plans. This approach is being phased in and will be complete by 2011.

A detailed explanation of the method is beyond the scope of the book and would be of doubtful value because the rules keep changing. Therefore, interested readers should go directly to CMS for information (a good place to start is the Web site http://www.cms.gov). Also, a thorough discussion of the method used is found in the *Essentials of Managed Health Care, Fifth Edition.*

Special Requirements for Medicare Advantage Plans

As noted earlier, the main MA participation requirement for MCOs is licensure by the state (though PSOs, under limited conditions, may not have to meet this requirement). CMS, however, has many additional requirements. These may vary between different types of plans to some degree, particularly between regional PPOs and local plans, and between coordinated care plans and PFFS or MSA plans. The most important of these requirements are described next.

Quality Standards

Each MA plan (other than PFFS and MSA plans) must have an ongoing quality improvement program. The organization must also encourage its providers to participate in CMS and DHHS quality improvement initiatives. In addition, each plan must have a chronic care improvement program (CCIP). The CCIP identifies enrollees with multiple or sufficiently severe chronic conditions who meet the criteria for participation in the program, and the program must have a mechanism for monitoring enrollees' participation. MA organizations are required to submit annual reports on their CCIP program to CMS.

Other quality requirements include the need to follow written policies and procedures that reflect current standards of medical practice when processing requests for initial or continued authorization of services (see Chapter 4). The plan must have in effect mechanisms to detect both underutilization and overutilization of services. A plan must be able to measure its performance using the measurement tools required by CMS. Plans report information on quality and outcomes measures to CMS so that CMS can provide this information to Medicare beneficiaries.

MA plans must also report the results of several standard reports and surveys, including:

- The Healthcare Effectiveness Data and Information Set (HEDIS), which provides information about service and quality
- The annual Consumer Assessment of Healthcare Providers and Systems (CAHPS) survey, a satisfaction and rating survey for enrollees and disenrollees
- The quarterly CAHPS Disenrollment Reasons Survey
- The Health Outcomes Survey (HOS)

Except for HEDIS and CAHPS, which are briefly discussed in Chapter 7, none of the tools listed above is covered in this book. For information about them, consult the *Essentials of Managed Health Care, Fifth Edition*, or go to http://www.cms.gov.

External Review

Coordinated care plans are subject to external review of the quality of care they render. The quality improvement organizations (QIOs, formerly peer review organizations) that are under contract to CMS to review the quality of care of hospitals in fee-for-service Medicare also review the quality of care among MA enrollees. The current approach to the role of the QIOs moves away from review of individual cases and toward a collaborative approach focusing on patterns of care. QIOs are also authorized to provide technical assistance to plans when they design their quality improvement projects and to evaluate the results of these projects. In addition, QIOs review complaints by MA enrollees about the quality of care in an MA plan. As in traditional Medicare, QIOs process beneficiary requests for review of hospital discharge decisions.

Deemed Compliance with Quality Requirements

Deemed compliance means that an MA organization may meet certain Medicare quality standards through accreditation by a private accrediting body. The accrediting organization must be approved by CMS, with approval subject to notice and comment in the Federal Register. The three accrediting organizations currently approved are the National Committee for Quality Assurance (NCQA), URAC (formerly called the Utilization Review Accreditation Commission, but it now uses only the initials), and the Accreditation Association for Ambulatory Health Care (AAAHC), all three of which are described in Chapter 7. The only requirements that may be deemed as met are quality assessment and performance improvement requirements, and confidentiality and accuracy of enrollee records requirements.

Limitations on Physician Incentive Plans

As noted in Chapter 3, a plan that has a physician incentive plan that places physicians at substantial financial risk (as defined in Medicare regulations[4]) for the care of Medicare or Medicaid enrollees must provide for continuous monitoring of the potential effects of the incentive plan on access or quality of care. This monitoring should include assessment of the results of surveys of enrollees and former enrollees using CAHPS, and the plan should review utilization data to identify patterns of possible underutilization of services that may be related to the incentive plan. Concerns identified as a result of this monitoring should be considered in development of the organization's focus areas for quality improvement projects. More detail on these limitations is provided in *Essentials of Managed Health Care, Fifth Edition*, or go to http://www.cms.gov.

Access Standards

With regard to access to care standards, the regulations have a number of requirements, including

- requiring unrestricted communication between patients and health care professionals through the prohibition of "gag" clauses;
- using the "prudent lay person" definition of what constitutes an emergency, the liability of the MA organization for the cost of such care, and a requirement to cover appropriate maintenance and poststabilization care after an emergency;
- covering out-of-area dialysis during an enrollee's temporary absence from the service area;
- limiting copayments for emergency services to no more than $50;
- specifying that the decision of the examining physician treating the individual enrollee prevails regarding when the enrollee may be considered stabilized for discharge or transfer (codification of existing policy);

---

[4] To oversimplify, physicians or physician groups are considered to be at substantial risk if over 25 percent of their potential payments are at risk.

- requiring plans to permit women enrollees to choose direct access to a women's health specialist within the network for women's routine and preventive health; and
- requiring that services be provided in a "culturally competent" manner (i.e., with sensitivity toward cultural, ethnic, and language differences).

Provider Protections

Providers are given certain protections against doing something that they believe goes against their conscience. These protections include

- a provision prohibiting discrimination against particular providers in selection of providers or payment or indemnification provisions solely on the basis of the provider's licensure status;
- appeal rights afforded to providers in the event of exclusion from a network; and
- a requirement that MA organizations consult with plan physicians regarding medical policy, quality, and medical management procedures.

The MA statute also permits a health care professional to refuse to provide advice, counseling, or referral for a service that the provider objects to on moral and religious grounds, as long as the MA organization provides notification to enrollees of the applicability of this provision. Finally, MA plans are required to meet the same prompt payment standards that apply to Medicare carriers and intermediaries in traditional Medicare with respect to the timeliness of payments made to noncontracted physicians and other providers for "clean" claims.

Member Appeals

Member appeals for Medicare are along the same lines as discussed in Chapters 5 and 7, but there are some specific differences. For MA plans, the steps of the appeals process include

- the determination by the MA plan (or a subcontracted entity);
- reconsideration by the MA plan, or, if the MA plan proposes a reconsideration decision adverse to the beneficiary, review of that decision by an external review entity under contract to CMS;
- review by an administrative law judge (for claims valued at $110 or more at the time of publication, an indexed amount subject to change each year) of the external review entity's decision if adverse to the beneficiary (but the MA plan is not entitled to appeal a decision by the external review entity when the decision is in favor of the beneficiary);

- review of the administrative law judge decision by the Departmental Appeals Board of the U.S. Department of Health and Human Services (a right available to members and to the MA plan); and
- judicial review in federal court for claims valued at $1,090 or more (as of the time of publication—this amount is also indexed).

The first-level determination is to be made by the MA plan within 14 days (or "as expeditiously as the enrollee's health condition requires" but no later than 14 days), and a reconsideration decision (by the MA plan or the review entity) is to be made within 30 days (with the same requirement for expeditious processing). For expedited appeals, the standard is that a decision must be rendered within 72 hours. QIOs also review beneficiary complaints, including beneficiary appeals about the appropriateness of a hospital discharge. Expedited time frames similar to those of traditional Medicare apply in such a case.

Grievances against an MA plan, as opposed to Medicare appeals, are subject to different standards. Beneficiaries must currently be afforded a right to "meaningful" grievance when the matter in dispute is an issue other than coverage or cost of an item or service that the MA organization is obligated to provide. CMS requires MA plans to provide data on the number of grievances and their results if an enrollee requests it.

Enrollment

Newly eligible Medicare beneficiaries may enroll in an MA plan as soon as they become eligible, as long as they also sign up for Medicare Part A and Part B benefits. Medicare beneficiaries who are Medicaid recipients may also enroll. The only Medicare beneficiaries not entitled to enroll (and to whom a plan must refuse enrollment under the law) are those who have end stage renal disease (ESRD), whether aged, disabled, or entitled to Medicare solely because of their disease. However, enrollees who acquire ESRD after enrollment in the plan may not be disenrolled because they have ESRD, and individuals who were enrolled as non-Medicare members of a plan who have ESRD may be retained as Medicare enrollees upon becoming eligible for Medicare. The one exception to the rule is that there can be special needs plans offered to individuals with ESRD who would not otherwise be entitled to enroll in an MA plan.

All MA plans, unless they are at capacity and unable to accept new members, hold an annual open enrollment that takes place from November 15 through December 31. During this "annual election period," beneficiaries receive comparative information on all their health care options, including traditional Medicare and its Medigap (supplemental coverage) options. They may elect new coverage and switch back and forth between MA and traditional Medicare, effective the following January. Newly eligible enrollees who do not choose an MA plan are deemed to have chosen the traditional Medicare option. If they choose not to have the drug benefit, even through a stand-alone PDP, they may have to pay higher premiums later should they decide they want it after all.

Between January 1 and March 31, individuals may make one election in or out of Medicare Advantage, but there can be no change in the person's election of drug coverage. After that, they are "locked in" to whatever option they chose for the remainder of the year, though certain exceptions do exist.

Finally, the MA plan must provide a description of benefits, called "evidence of coverage," which includes information on benefits and exclusions; the number, mix, and distribution of plan providers; out-of-network and out-of-area coverage; emergency coverage (how it is defined and how to gain access to emergency care, including use of 911 services); prior authorization or other review requirements; grievances and appeals; and a description of the plan's quality assurance program. On request, the organization must provide information on utilization control practices, the number and disposition of appeals and grievances, and a summary description of physician compensation.

Sales and Marketing

Except for employer-sponsored MA plans (not discussed in this book), MA plans market and sell their products to individual Medicare beneficiaries, and a beneficiary's decision to join an MCO is based on purely personal reasons. CMS has created many rules for market conduct, however, such as the following:

- The MCO must market throughout the entire service area in a nondiscriminatory manner.
- All marketing materials, including membership and enrollment materials, must be approved by CMS before use (though there is a time limit on CMS's review process, and model language exists as well).
- Prospective enrollees must be given sufficient descriptive materials to allow them to make an informed decision regarding enrollment.
- Prospective enrollees must be given a summary of benefits form that uses standard definitions of benefits and a standardized format.

Some sales and marketing activities are explicitly prohibited, and an MA plan that engages in these activities is subject to fines, suspension of their ability to enroll new members, or other sanctions. Examples of sales and marketing activities that are prohibited by CMS are

- door-to-door solicitation,
- discriminatory marketing (e.g., avoiding low-income areas),
- misleading marketing or misrepresentation,
- offering monetary incentives as an inducement to enroll, and
- completing any portion of the enrollment application for a prospective enrollee.

Corporate Compliance

Corporate compliance activities are directed toward (1) ensuring that the organization conforms to legal and regulatory requirements and (2) preventing and detecting illegal behavior. Corporate compliance applies to all MCOs under a variety of laws and regulations, including Medicare. Because there is considerable overlap, it is permissible and practical to combine the corporate compliance activities for most or all of the different laws and regulations into one overall compliance function.

For MA plans specifically, CMS, through the Office of the Inspector General (OIG), has created corporate compliance guidelines that an MA plan must follow. The full set of corporate compliance requirements is rather complex, but in general, for an MA corporate compliance program to be effective, the following are required:

- Creation of a special compliance committee
- Designation of a corporate compliance officer
- Creation of standards of conduct for employees
- Creation of policies and procedures specifically designed to ensure compliance with MA rules
- Special training for employees
- Employee surveys that focus on compliance issues
- A "hotline" for employees to report violations of MA rules
- Exit interviews of employees in which possible rule violations are inquired about
- Audits of compliance
- Screening for individuals or entities barred from participation in federal programs (applies to employees, providers, and vendors)
- Creation of an internal investigation program that focuses on MA rule violations

MEDICAID

At the same time that Medicare was created in 1965, an additional program was created to provide health insurance coverage for low-income individuals—Medicaid. Beyond covering individuals, Medicaid also provides major subsidies to safety net hospitals to provide uncompensated care to millions of uninsured persons. Unlike

Medicare, Medicaid is administered by the states, though half of the funding comes from the federal government. Policies, rules, and regulations pertaining to eligibility, coverage, payment, and services vary from state to state. National legislation, including the Americans with Disabilities Act, welfare reform legislation, the BBA, the State Children's Health Insurance Program (SCHIP), and the MMA have also had, and continue to have, a direct impact on Medicaid.

Medicaid provides coverage primarily for three groups:

1. Low-income individuals, mostly healthy women and children, who make up 70 percent of Medicaid enrollees.
2. Aged and younger persons who have a chronic illness or condition and are disabled, who make up the second largest group.
3. Institutionalized individuals, who make up the third group. This is really a subset of the second group. This population includes aged persons needing nursing home care who are either impoverished at the time of their admission or become so during their stay, and persons in specialized facilities for the developmentally disabled or mentally retarded.

The second two groups, despite representing a minority of the Medicaid enrollees, are responsible for the vast majority of Medicaid costs. It is the first group, however, that has historically been the primary focus of Medicaid managed care, because these individuals are most similar to the commercial population and therefore more easily integrated into managed care programs. That focus may be changing.

Background and History

Like Medicare, Medicaid was operated as a fee-for-service program, and providers billed Medicaid for services rendered. Physicians are not required to participate in the Medicaid program (i.e., agree to accept Medicaid reimbursement as payment in full), and many do not. Hospitals are not required to participate unless they are nonprofit; however, almost all hospitals participate regardless because even though Medicaid pays them less than it costs to provide care, it is better than not getting paid at all.

Because Medicaid consumes ever increasing portions of each state's budget, states are continually looking for ways to control the cost of the program. For the most part, to achieve this goal, states have used the strategy of paying very low fees to providers. Although partially successful as a way of moderating cost increases, this strategy has also had the unintended effect of obstructing access to care; many providers, physicians in particular, are unwilling to accept Medicaid patients in return for low levels of reimbursement.

In the early 1980s, a few states, led by Arizona and a few counties in California, began to explore whether Medicaid could use selective contracting strategies with subsets of providers or with prepaid health plans (early vintage HMOs; see Chapter 2) to obtain guaranteed access to reputable providers at more predictable and, ideally, more manageable future costs. Other states soon followed suit, including some, like Utah and Michigan, that chose to contract with individual primary care physicians as "primary care case managers" (PCCMs) because they had few or no willing prepaid health plans. By the end of the 1980s, enrollment in managed care arrangements approached three million, or about 15 percent of Medicaid beneficiaries. Enrollment jumped in the mid-1990s when states chose, with encouragement from federal authorities, to devise a variety of reform strategies that included combinations of managed care and eligibility expansions. Soon, more than half of all states had some managed care initiatives. In all cases, however, the state needed special permission from the federal government to create such programs.

By 1997, the federal government extended to states the opportunity to routinely require low-income beneficiaries to obtain Medicaid benefits through choice-restricting prepaid health plans or PCCM programs. This promoted further expansion, and by the end of the 1990s, nearly 20 million individuals—which is over 50 percent of the Medicaid population—was in some kind of managed care arrangement. During this period, nearly all managed care enrollees were low-income women and children.

In the early 2000s, Medicaid enrollment continued to grow, with over 40 states offering some form of managed care and several beginning to test managed care for disabled and chronically ill beneficiaries. By 2005, Medicaid managed enrollment totaled nearly 30 million beneficiaries, or 63 percent of the total population in the program. Approximately 80 percent of these persons are enrolled in fully capitated health plans[5] (though selected services are carved out in some states), and the remainder are in PCCM programs (particularly in rural states).

Currently, there are a variety of Medicaid managed care programs. In some states, commercial HMOs offer services. Most states also have commercially operated Medicaid-only plans that look much like traditional HMOs, though they also have capabilities specific to meeting the needs of Medicaid beneficiaries. Such commercially operated plans may be part of a traditional multi-line health insurer or MCO, they may be part of a national for-profit company that specializes in

---

[5] In this context, it is the health plan that is capitated, not necessarily the participating providers who may be reimbursed under any of the mechanisms described in Chapter 3.

Medicaid, or they may be locally owned and operated. Locally owned and operated plans may be for-profit or not-for-profit and in some cases are owned or sponsored by provider organizations. Finally, a few states actually run their own managed care programs. These state-run programs may look like HMOs, but more frequently they are PCCM plans. In the PCCM model, Medicaid members use primary care physicians to coordinate care, but other HMO features, such as financial risk sharing, are absent.

Operational Issues for Medicaid Health Plans

State Medicaid agencies employ multiple approaches to selecting which plans will be offered to their beneficiaries. Some states set participation qualifications for interested plans—including payment rates—and select all who meet them. Others require periodic bidding and may award a limited number of contracts. How participating plans are paid also varies among states. States have become more detailed and demanding in their contracting with health plans, including key requirements like provider network access standards, customer service standards and obligations, performance data submission, external reviews, and many others.

In all cases in which a Medicaid MCO accepts risk, the state capitates the plan, but how that capitation amount is calculated varies. In some states, only age and sex (and often urban vs. rural as well) are used to adjust payments, whereas some states are now experimenting with adjusting payments based on how ill a Medicaid member is, providing higher capitation payments if the plan has sicker than average members, or lower payments if members are healthier on average; this approach is similar to the one being phased in for MA plans noted earlier.

Most states currently mandate (i.e., require) enrollment in managed care for low-income women and children. A few states do this for other populations, but in most states where disabled or chronically ill are eligible for managed care plans, enrollment is voluntary or, if mandatory, liberal exemptions are permitted. However, one of the most frustrating administrative concerns for Medicaid managed care plans is the high rate of member turnover commonly referred to as "churning." Tying enrollment to Medicaid eligibility means that plan members drop in and out based on fluctuations in their income and assets, or on whether they even remember to reapply for benefits that must be periodically recertified.

Medicaid agencies carefully regulate marketing by health plans, typically relying on independent enrollment brokers to orchestrate the plan choice process and prohibiting plans from doing direct marketing. For persons who do not make a plan choice, the state agency automatically assigns them to a health plan.

Medicaid managed care is a demanding line of business, requiring plans to serve populations with complex medical and social needs and forcing them to develop provider networks of considerable diversity—both in terms of service capabilities and cultural competencies. Cultural diversity is a highly important issue in Medicaid, including the need to accommodate non-English-speaking individuals. Because of the low educational levels prevalent in some Medicaid populations, materials that explain the program have to be written in easy-to-understand language. Transportation services, proactive outreach, attentiveness to physical and social environmental factors, and increasing cultural competency are all areas in which plans must develop proficiency to have positive, sustained impacts on their members. The concentrations of high-risk pregnancies in this population, as well as persistence of chronic conditions like asthma, diabetes, depression, and substance abuse, require well-planned interventions to promote member well-being and to achieve cost-effective outcomes.

In some states, arrangements are in place for certain services to be carved out and provided separately from the basic health plan, as well as specialized models for behavioral health and special needs populations (e.g. foster care, developmentally delayed children). Some states carve out the pharmacy benefits, which are then administered by a separate pharmacy benefits management program. Several states are now employing disease management and intensive care management (see Chapter 4) for certain beneficiaries.

States monitor the activities of Medicaid MCOs in much the same way that the federal government monitors the activities of MA plans. One particularly important measurement tool is a Medicaid-specific version of HEDIS. Other types of measurements may also be used by states, though HEDIS remains the standard that is most prevalent.

Some states have pushed plans to move into pay-for-performance arrangements (see Chapter 3) and, in a few instances, to extend these models to network providers. By working through plans and placing performance reporting requirements on them, states can exert more influence on providers than most chose to do when they dealt with providers directly. Though many states focused almost exclusively on managing costs at the outset, more and more of them are shifting their emphasis to managing care, both as a way of improving quality in response to their critics and as a way of better controlling long-term costs.

Special Needs Plans for Dual Medicare/Medicaid Beneficiaries

As noted earlier, the MMA authorized the creation of SNPs to serve persons who had dual eligibility for Medicare and Medicaid. Among the "duals" are both low-income and frail seniors, and younger adults with disabling chronic illnesses and disabilities. As a whole, the seven million dual eligible individuals represent about 18 percent of its 40 million enrollees, but they are nearly twice as expensive as other Medicare beneficiaries. For Medicaid, though, this 14 percent of the total 50 million enrollees represents about 40 percent of expenditures enrollees, primarily because of their needs for long-term supports and services. The number of these newly created plans has grown rapidly, but few have yet developed contracts for complete Medicaid services, and even fewer have developed plans for long-term care services. Nevertheless, SNPs are expected to grow in the future.

CONCLUSION

Medicare and Medicaid, as entitlement health care programs at the federal and state levels, together represent enormous expenditures of tax dollars. Medicare, by implementing managed care, has been able to improve its health care benefits while keeping costs reasonable. The creation of a new drug benefit has also provided greater benefits to those who enroll in that program, and managing this benefit has become a major area of focus for managed care. State Medicaid programs have successfully used managed care to control costs, improve access, and enhance the coordination of care, which explains why most states have incorporated managed care into their Medicaid programs. Because Medicare and Medicaid are government programs and have widely different characteristics, MCOs that undertake to serve Medicare and Medicaid populations must be prepared to focus or modify their operations to meet the programs' special requirements.

Substantial sections in this chapter are adapted from C. J. Zarabozo and S. Lindenberg, "Health Plans and Medicare," and from R. Hurley and S. Somers, "Medicaid Managed Care," in *The Essentials of Managed Health Care,* 5th edition, ed. P. R. Kongstvedt (Sudbury, MA: Jones & Bartlett, Publishers, 2007).

7

Regulation and Accreditation in Managed Care

LEARNING OBJECTIVES

- Understand the basic issues involved with state regulation of managed care
- Understand the limited continuation of coverage benefit under COBRA
- Understand the key components of the Health Insurance Portability and Accountability Act
- Understand the key components of the Employee Retirement Income Security Act
- Understand the key components of external accreditation of managed care organizations

Managed care is heavily regulated, but regulation is far from uniform. For most aspects of managed care, the states are responsible for regulating managed care organizations (MCOs). States do so under a wide variety of laws and regulations, and these are applied to almost every aspect of how an MCO operates. Laws and regulations not only differ between states, but also usually differ depending on the type of MCO being regulated. However, the states have for many years made efforts to bring their respective laws closer into alignment to each other.

One critical factor is that state regulation generally applies only to that part of an MCO's business for which medical services are insured by an MCO (i.e., services for which the MCO accepts the risk for medical expenses). If an employer retains the risk for medical expenses and the MCO simply provides administrative services, the state has significantly less authority, and the provision of medical services are regulated under a federal law entitled the Employee Retirement Income Security Act (ERISA). As a practical matter, most MCOs, because they have insured and self-insured accounts, are regulated by both the states and under ERISA, but in different ways. However, as will be discussed later, some elements of state regulation do apply to the provision of medical care even when covered through self-insured employers.

In 1996, the Health Insurance Portability and Accountability Act (HIPAA) was signed into law. It placed requirements and regulatory responsibilities on almost all elements of the health care system, including providers and MCOs, regardless of any other state or federal regulation.

This chapter briefly describes the regulation of MCOs by the states and the requirements set by HIPAA and ERISA. The chapter also briefly addresses formal accreditation programs for MCOs, programs that are increasingly being relied on by state and federal agencies and employers. The reader should bear in mind that laws and accreditation standards are always changing and that only very up-to-date sources should be relied on for information about accreditation and the regulations that pertain to MCOs.

STATE REGULATION

MCOs may be regulated by more than one state agency. In almost all cases, the department of insurance (DOI) regulates health maintenance organizations (HMOs), although some exceptions exist (e.g., in California, HMOs are regulated separately). In many states, the department of health (DOH) also regulates HMOs. Insurance regulators assume principal responsibility for the financial aspects of HMO operations and, in many states, for external review of adverse benefit determinations. Health regulators focus on quality-of-care issues, utilization patterns, and the ability of participating providers to deliver adequate care. Risk-bearing preferred provider organizations (PPOs)—PPOs that also provide health insurance coverage—are generally regulated by the DOI, whereas non-risk-bearing PPOs—PPOs that are only a network of contracted providers working with different insurance companies—may be regulated by the DOH, if they are regulated at all.

The National Association of Insurance Commissioners (NAIC), which represents insurance departments in the 50 states and the U.S. territories, created the HMO Model Act in 1972 as a model for legislation authorizing the establishment of HMOs and provides for an ongoing regulatory monitoring system. This model act, either in whole or in part, has now been enacted by 30 states and the District of Columbia. The remaining states also have adopted laws regulating HMOs, but these laws are not always based on the NAIC's HMO Model Act. The NAIC has also created other model acts for PPOs and utilization review organizations, as well as for issues such as network adequacy, provider contracting and payment terms, privacy, external review, financial solvency, and so forth. None of these model acts has the force of law, but each may be used by states in creating their own laws and regulations.

Licensure

The most important type of state regulation of risk-bearing MCOs is licensure. The license, often termed a certificate of authority (COA), sets out the requirements that the MCO must meet to do business in the state. These requirements are laid out in the model act or in one of many model acts that apply to specific functions (quality management, for example). The many requirements for licensure include:

- Financial solvency (i.e., the MCO must have sufficient money to reliably pay claims)
- An adequate network
- Adequate access to care, including uninterrupted access to emergency services
- An acceptable utilization management program
- An acceptable quality management program
- An acceptable member grievance program (the model act has been modified to make it more like ERISA in this regard and is discussed later in this chapter)
- A provider credentialing verification system
- Adequate information for members
- Benefits plans that meet state requirements
- Proper forms for groups
- Proper forms for enrollees
- Conversion rights for disenrolling members (i.e., some members who lose group coverage have the right to convert to an individual policy)

The exact nature of these requirements varies depending on the type of MCO (e.g., HMO or PPO), and some requirements may not apply under certain conditions (e.g., a non-risk-bearing PPO).

In addition to granting a license to an MCO, the DOI monitors the MCO's performance on a regular basis. For monitoring purposes, the state requires the MCO to provide quarterly financial reports and audited annual financial statements. If DOI officials believe that the MCO is not performing well (e.g., if it appears to be running low on money), they may intensify their scrutiny. In the most extreme circumstances, such as when bankruptcy appears imminent, the state DOI may even seize control of the MCO to protect the interests of the covered members.

A third-party administrator (TPA) is an organization that administers group benefits and claims for a self-funded company or group. It usually does not assume any insurance risk, but neither is it considered a self-funded health plan under ERISA. Therefore, about two-thirds of the states require licensure of TPAs, but about one-third exempt TPAs from state licensure if they administer only single-employer, self-funded plans. State TPA laws typically govern the following:

- The TPA's written agreement with each insurer (which must include a statement of duties)
- The payment methodology
- The maintenance and disclosure of records
- Insurer responsibilities, such as the determination of benefit levels
- The TPA's fiduciary obligations (e.g., in the collecting of charges and premiums)
- The issuance of TPA licenses and grounds for suspension or revocation
- The filing of annual reports
- The payment of fees

In addition to licensing health plans, many states require additional licensure or certification for utilization management activities that an MCO or TPA undertakes. Under the NAIC's Utilization Review Model Act, HMOs, PPOs, freestanding medical management organizations, and other health care organizations that are subject to state regulation and provide or perform utilization review services are required to:

- Use documented clinical review criteria based on sound clinical evidence
- Ensure that qualified health professionals administer the utilization review program
- Abide by strict time limits for utilization review decisions

The model act prohibits compensation arrangements that encourage utilization review staff to make inappropriate determinations and provides for a process of appealing adverse decisions.

Any Willing Provider

As discussed in Chapters 1 and 2, the creation of selective provider panels is a cornerstone of MCO operations. Many states, however, have enacted "any willing provider" (AWP) laws that prevent MCOs from selectively contracting with a limited group of providers. In most instances, AWP laws apply to specific categories of providers, such as pharmacists, rather than across the board to include all providers. Such laws generally require an MCO to accept into its network any provider willing to meet the terms and conditions of the MCO's contract, as long as that provider also meets credentialing requirements as discussed in Chapter 3.

By the end of 2005, approximately half of the states had adopted AWP laws affecting MCOs. Many of these laws are limited to pharmacists (requiring MCOs to accept into the plan's network nonparticipating pharmacists willing to meet the MCO's terms and conditions), but in some of these states, HMOs receive full or partial exemptions from such open pharmacy requirements. In some states, AWP laws apply to physicians and other types of providers (e.g., chiropractors) as well. State AWP laws have been legally challenged on the basis of federal preemption under ERISA. However, in 2003, the U.S. Supreme Court, in a unanimous decision, found that a Kentucky AWP law was not preempted by ERISA and therefore was allowed to stand. As a result, AWP laws can be enforced by the state even for self-funded plans.

Regulation of Insured Business

Most state laws and regulations apply to MCOs that are at risk for medical expenses and are not just providing administrative services. Some of the more common types are described next. The creation (and the rare removal) of these laws and regulations is influenced by politics, and thus they differ widely from state to state. As noted, except for AWP laws, the provision of medical services by self-insured employers is governed by the provisions of ERISA (discussed in a later section) and is generally outside the scope of these laws and regulations. In fact, many employers self-insure primarily to avoid having their benefits plans subject to these laws and regulations.

Benefits Plans and Premium Rates

Every state requires MCOs to file benefits plans and premium rates. Some states require MCOs to obtain approval before offering benefits plans, and others simply require notification. State rules that determine how MCOs may create premium rates also vary (for example, as noted in Chapter 5, community rating may be required for small groups). It is common for an MCO to file a benefits plan in which some options are offered to enrollees, such as three different levels of copayment for physician visits. In filing the benefits plan, the MCO indicates what the options are.

Mandated Benefits

Most states have laws mandating certain benefits (e.g., mental health benefits, substance abuse benefits, infertility benefits, and so forth). If a benefit has been mandated, all MCOs and health insurance companies must offer that benefit in their insured products. Some states have many mandated benefits, others have relatively few. Some state laws mandating benefits also contain provisions directing how the benefits are to be applied. In the most common example, a state law might set a mandatory length of stay, such as 2 days, for the delivery of a baby, in which case an MCO may not discharge a newborn and mother in less than 2 days, unless the patient herself requests it.

Provider-MCO Relationships

In addition to AWP laws discussed earlier, some states have laws regulating other aspects of the relationship between MCOs and providers. Prompt payment laws, which require MCOs to process claims and pay providers within a set amount of time, are the most common example. Some states also have laws that require an MCO or insurer to pay a provider directly even if the provider does not have a contract with the MCO. Laws may also exist that regulate conditions under which an MCO may or may not terminate a provider from its network.

Provider Access

Access to certain types of providers has been legally protected in some states. For instance, laws giving women the right to access OB/GYNs directly without having to go through a primary care provider are common. A few states have also passed laws allowing direct access to other types of providers, such as chiropractors, and a few have passed laws requiring an MCO to create a "standing authorization" for specialty physician services for certain clinical conditions. As for access to emergency services, most states require an MCO to use a "prudent layperson" standard in determining whether to pay for emergency care. In other words, if a normal nonclinically trained person would have been convinced that a true emergency existed, then the MCO must pay for the care.

External Appeals

All states have regulations about how a member may appeal a denial of coverage for medical services. In 2000, the U.S. Department of Labor (DOL), which administers ERISA, put out its regulation establishing standards for benefit claims procedures of employee benefits plans. It set out specific requirements governing the time periods for making benefit determinations and deciding appeals, notice and disclosure requirements, standards of review, and the use of arbitration or other dispute resolution procedures (ERISA is discussed later in this chapter). MCOs that contract with employers to provide insured health benefits as well as the administration of health benefits for ERISA plans are subject to both state law requirements and the DOL claim procedures rule.

After the DOL issued its regulation, the NAIC revisited the Grievance Procedure Model and amended it to more closely follow the federal requirements. However, the model continues to contain requirements in addition to those under the federal regulation. For example, the Grievance Procedure Model gives an enrollee the option of a second level of internal appeal, whereas the federal regulation permits, but does not require, an MCO to establish a second appeal level.

Although state-level policies may differ, the right to an external review generally applies to denials of coverage that are based on medical necessity criteria or a determination that the services are experimental or investigational. In addition, these policies often contain provisions such as the following:

- The internal appeals process must be completed before the external review can be initiated.
- The plan must select an independent review entity from a list approved by the state or by a state official (typically the insurance commissioner).
- The external review entity must not be subject to a conflict of interest.
- The plan must pay the costs of the external review process.
- The external review entity's decision is to be binding on the plan.

Privacy

In recent years, state laws protecting the privacy of health care information have become popular. HIPAA also has provisions protecting the privacy and security of health information, but it allows states to pass stricter laws and regulations. HIPAA is discussed later in this chapter.

Solvency Standards and Insolvency Protections

To prevent MCO financial insolvencies (i.e., bankruptcy) and protect consumers and providers against the effects of insolvencies that do occur, the model act establishes specific financial capital, reserve, and deposit requirements that all MCOs must meet. Before a COA is even issued to an HMO, for example, an initial net worth of $3 million is required. After issuance, a minimum net worth must be maintained by the HMO equal to the greater of $2.5 million or an amount equal to a percentage of medical benefits payments already being made (e.g., enough cash to pay for 3 months' worth of claims for insured business). This net worth is also referred to as surplus. The HMO Model Act also requires a minimum deposit of $1 million with the state insurance department, though that deposit is considered the MCO's asset.

The NAIC adopted a more flexible approach to determining how much capital MCOs must have, replacing the idea of a percentage of claims already being paid. It is called risk-based capital (RBC), and it recognizes that financial surplus requirements will vary from one MCO to another based on the specific nature of the MCO's business. For example, the RBC formula permits state regulators to assess the specific risk profile of individual MCOs and give credit for provider contracting mechanisms (such as capitation and withholds) that reduce the financial risk borne by an MCO. The RBC formula also takes other elements into account, such as the risk that an affiliated entity could cost an MCO money, that premiums may not be high enough to pay claims, that an MCO's own insurance coverage is inadequate, and so forth.

As discussed in Chapter 3, most states also require HMOs to include "hold harmless" clauses in their provider contracts. In situations in which the HMO fails to pay for covered medical care, such clauses prohibit providers from seeking collection from the enrollees. Several states also require that HMOs enter into reinsurance arrangements to cover liabilities in the event that the MCO becomes insolvent. In addition, most states require solvent HMOs in the market to provide coverage to enrollees of the insolvent HMO. Such requirements are less likely to be applied to non-HMO MCOs.

Many states also require PPOs, particularly risk-bearing PPOs, to meet requirements relating to solvency and insolvency protections. Some have established PPO-specific requirements, such as posting a bond equal to 10 percent of the PPO's estimated aggregate reimbursement, whereas others require that risk-bearing PPOs abide by the solvency requirements applicable to HMOs or indemnity insurers. This latter approach has led to increasing use of RBC solvency standards for PPOs as more and more states adopt the RBC model.

Health Plan Liability

In all states, MCOs can be held liable based on the same principles of liability applied to hospitals—including vicarious liability and direct corporate liability—for such acts as the negligent hiring and supervision of physicians, failure to provide adequate facilities and equipment, and consumer fraud and misrepresentation. Whether for profit or not for profit, MCOs are still corporations.

In the past, a particular provision of ERISA limited the legal liability of insurance companies and health plans and effectively prevented enrollees from obtaining significant punitive damage awards from tort suits (i.e., lawsuits claiming damages). If a health plan or an insurance company did not act in bad faith, the most that a plaintiff could recover was the insurance benefit itself. Certainly, some lawsuits resulted in large damage awards, but such awards were difficult to obtain. Some states have passed laws that increase the liability of health plans and insurance companies and make them subject to punitive damages in lawsuits. The issue of liability is the subject of intense ongoing debate at the federal level, because ERISA is a federal law.

Multistate Operations

MCOs operating in more than one state must comply with the regulations of each state. It is usual for a state to require "foreign" MCOs (i.e., MCOs licensed in a different state) to meet the same requirements that apply to "domestic" MCOs. It is also possible for a state to require foreign MCOs to register to do business under the appropriate foreign corporation law and appoint an agent in the state for receipt of legal notifications.

Some states permit regulators to accept financial reports and other information from a foreign MCO's state of origin, often referred to as the state of domicile. The NAIC also has established guidelines for coordinating examinations of MCOs licensed in more than one state. The coordinated examination is called for by the MCO's state of domicile; other states where the MCO operates are encouraged to participate. Occasionally, regulations in one state may hinder the operations of an MCO licensed in another state.

Historically, group insurance policies were usually subject only to the laws of the state of issuance (i.e., the state where the policies were originally issued), but this has been changing. It is now common for a state to require that any state resident covered under a group health policy issued in a different state receive the same coverage that would have been required had the group policy been issued within the state.

THE HEALTH INSURANCE PORTABILITY AND ACCOUNTABILITY ACT

HIPAA, a highly significant federal act passed in 1996 by a Republican congress and signed into law by a Democratic president, represents the first direct intrusion of the federal government into the regulation of insurance. As noted in the previous section, states regulate insurance while the federal government regulates self-insured benefits plans, with the exception of some ERISA regulations around appeal rights. The provisions of HIPAA apply equally to insured and self-insured health benefits plans. However, HIPAA does not preempt state law provisions that are more stringent than the corresponding provisions in HIPAA, except in one area—electronic transaction standards and code sets (discussed later in this section).

Portability and Access

HIPAA establishes standards for group health plans and group health insurance coverage that are intended to enhance access to health coverage. For HIPAA, a group health plan is an employer- or union-sponsored employee benefit plan (as defined in ERISA) that provides medical care through insurance, reimbursement, or otherwise. The health insurance issuer might be an insurance company, an insurance service organization, an HMO, or most any type of risk-bearing MCO.

HIPAA addresses the issue of preexisting medical conditions for group medical insurance. It states that for a group policy, enrollment cannot be denied to individuals with preexisting medical conditions, nor can waiting periods be applied to the provision of services for these individuals based on their having these conditions. HIPAA also prohibits charging different premium rates to people within the same health benefits plan based solely on their medical conditions. HIPAA does not actually require any particular benefits (with a few exceptions noted later in this section). In other words, HIPAA does not dictate plan benefit design but does ensure greater access to group insurance benefits, whatever they might be.

HIPAA contains provisions about guaranteed renewability of group health insurance, as well as certain forms of health insurance portability. With regard to renewability, if a small employer (i.e., an employer with between 2 and 50 employees) has an insured health benefits plan with an insurance carrier, the employer has the right to renew its coverage with the carrier. In fact, HIPAA goes so far as to require insurance companies to guarantee access to their most common small-group products to any small employers who seek them. It does not say anything about the cost of that insurance, however, though most states do have laws and regulations about premiums in the small-group market.

There are actually two separate federal laws (and scattered differing state laws) that provide individuals with the right to extend their health insurance coverage with an insurer if they lose their group health coverage and do not have any other group health benefits plan available to them. Certain conditions must be met for this provision to apply, however. For example, individuals cannot decide not to enroll in their group's health insurance plan and then later change their mind when they need care. They must enroll when they have the opportunity to do so and not wait until they think they will need the coverage.

The Consolidated Omnibus Reconciliation Act (COBRA) requires an employer with 20 or more employees in a group medical benefits plan to offer terminated employees the opportunity to purchase continuation of health care coverage under the employer's medical plan for an 18-month period (longer if the employees are disabled) or until eligible for another group health benefits plan. The same right to continue coverage (up to 36 months) is also available to an ex-spouse or surviving spouse in the event of divorce or death, as long as the ex- or surviving spouse does not have access to group health insurance on his or her own. The premium cost cannot exceed the cost of the premium paid by the employer (plus an additional 2 percent administrative fee), but the individual must pay the entire premium because the employer does not contribute to the cost of the insurance. Someone who qualifies for a COBRA extension of coverage must apply for it within 60 days of qualifying.

HIPAA guarantees an additional form of individual portability of health insurance. This means that regardless of health status, individuals who have maintained continuous coverage and who then lose coverage under a group health plan may purchase coverage in the individual purchaser market. To be eligible for individual coverage under HIPAA, a person must

- have 18 or more months of aggregate creditable coverage (the most recent coverage must have come from a group health plan, government plan, or church plan or have been health insurance coverage linked to any such plan);
- be ineligible for group health coverage, Medicare, or Medicaid;
- lack other health insurance coverage;
- have not been terminated from his or her most recent prior coverage for nonpayment of premiums or fraud; and
- have elected and exhausted COBRA coverage or similar state-mandated continuation coverage if he or she was eligible for it.

Nothing in HIPAA controls the amount of premium that a health insurer may charge for individual coverage, so such policies are almost always very expensive. The act includes specific details about when enrollment must occur and what circumstances must be obtained for an individual to gain the protected access to health insurance that the act provides.

Specific Clinical Conditions Addressed in HIPAA

Three clinical conditions were addressed though amendments or Acts to the original act. The Newborns' and Mothers' Health Protection Act of 1996 mandates a minimum 48-hour length of stay for normal vaginal deliveries and a 96-hour length of stay for cesarean sections. These minimum lengths of stay are voluntary, of course, and a woman can ask to be discharged sooner if she desires. But a health plan may not refuse authorization of coverage for less than these minimums.

The Mental Health Parity Act of 1996 requires that the aggregate lifetime dollar limits and annual dollar limits for mental health benefits and medical-surgical benefits be equal. Ironically, it does not actually require benefits plans to offer mental health benefits, nor does it require the same levels of copayment or coinsurance if it does; it only requires the same lifetime and annual limits. The issue of mental health benefits within group health insurance remains a contentious topic of political debate even as this is being written.

The Women's Health and Cancer Rights Act of 1998 requires that group health plans, as well as health insurance that covers medical and surgical benefits for mastectomies, also provide coverage for (1) all stages of breast reconstruction, (2) surgery and reconstruction of the other breast to produce a symmetrical appearance, and (3) prostheses and physical complications of mastectomy. The act does not change any requirements a health plan may have regarding levels of coverage for using contracting versus noncontracting providers, however.

Administrative Simplification

The section of HIPAA that concerns administrative simplification is considered the most important section of the law. The goal of this section is to reduce the administrative costs and burden in health care, standardize certain data elements, and protect the privacy of an individual's health information. All the section's provisions are currently in force, but HIPAA also provides a mechanism for continually updating exactly what is contained in those provisions. The four basic aspects of administrative simplification are transactions and code sets, the national provider identifier, privacy of medical information, and security of medical information.

Administrative simplification under HIPAA does not just apply to health plans. There is a long list of "covered entities" that must comply with HIPAA. Examples include hospitals, all types of licensed health care providers, pharmacies, claim clearinghouses, and so forth. HIPAA also addresses requirements for "business associates" of covered entities, which are companies or individuals who provide services to a covered entity and must therefore comply with the same requirements as the covered entity, though it is the covered entity's responsibility to make sure that happens. For example, a company that runs a health plan's computer system must agree to comply with privacy and security requirements.

Transactions and Code Sets

The transactions in question are electronic transfers of data between providers and payers, among others, and the code sets are the definitions of the data. Prior to HIPAA, the transactions and code sets were not standardized to any great degree. The goal of the administrative simplification section of HIPAA was to create a single, uniform national standard for electronic transactions and thereby reduce errors, make the transactions easier and cheaper, and encourage their use by all parties. The transaction and code set provisions in HIPAA completely preempt state law. These standards are highly technical, and a sense of that is provided by simply listing what they are.

Electronic Transaction Standards. For transactions other than pharmacy claims, the transaction standards are those of the X12 (sometimes referred to as X12N) standards of the American National Standards Institute (ANSI). When the mandated standards went into effect in 2002, version 4010 of the X12 standards was the one chosen. Newer versions now exist, but because of the need to maintain stability in standards so as to encourage adoption, the 4010 versions remain the standard at the time of publication. Migration to the 5010 version is expected to occur at some point in the relatively near future. For pharmacy claims, the designated standards are those of the National Council for Prescription Drug Programs (NCPDP), Batch Standard Implementation Guide, and Telecommunication Standard Implementation Guide. Not all standards required under HIPAA have been finalized, however; for example, at the time of publication, the standard for the claims attachment[1] was proposed (but not officially designated) to be the 4050 version of ANSI 275 combined with the Clinical Architecture Document (CDA) standards

---

[1] A claims attachment is additional clinical information that an MCO might need to process a claim; such information is now usually provided by paper copy.

from Health Level 7 (HL7), whereas the standard for First Report of Injury had not yet been proposed at all. The electronic transaction standards under HIPAA are listed in Table 7–1.

The standards themselves are subject to periodic updating. Under HIPAA, Designated Standards Maintenance Organizations (DSMOs) are charged with making recommendations to the federal government regarding updates to existing standards, as well as the addition of new standards. The following organizations are considered DSMOs under HIPAA:

1. Accredited Standards Committee X12 (also known as the American National Standards Institute–ANSI)
2. Dental Content Committee of the American Dental Association
3. Health Level Seven (HL7)
4. National Council for Prescription Drug Programs (NCPDP)
5. National Uniform Billing Committee
6. National Uniform Claim Committee

Code Set Standards. Code sets refer to the types of standardized codes that must be used in the transactions as they apply to different types of clinical services, and they are very extensive. The standardized code sets required under HIPAA are listed in Exhibit 7–1.

All these heavily used code sets have been in existence for quite a while, though with periodic updating and modifications. At the time of publication, consideration is being given via the DSMOs to updating ICD–9 to ICD–10 (which would also incorporate many of the codes that are currently covered by HCPCS). The ICD–10 code set is approximately 10 times the size of the ICD–9 set and considerably more complex, and it will require considerable modifications to provider and payer systems (both commercial and governmental); one date being discussed for implementation is 2012, but when it will actually take place is not known. The AMA is currently undertaking a project to develop the CPT–5 code set, but there is no discussion at the time of publication as to when that would be generally adopted.

National Identifiers

HIPAA mandates that uniform identifiers be used by all health plans and providers. A national employer identifier is also addressed in HIPAA but is not a priority. HIPAA originally also addressed a uniform patient identifier, but that provision was permanently taken out of consideration because of privacy con-

Table 7–1 HIPAA Standardized Electronic Transactions

Transaction	Standard
Provider claims submission	ANSI X12-837 (different versions exist for institutional, professional, and dental)
Pharmacy claims	NCPDP
Eligibility	ANSI X12-270 (inquiry)
	ANSI X12-271 (response)
Claim status	ANSI X12-276 (inquiry)
	ANSI X12-277 (response)
Provider referral certification and authorization	ANSI X12-278
Health care payment to provider, with remittance advice	ANSI X12-835
Enrollment and disenrollment in health plan*	ANSI X12-834
Claims attachment (additional clinical information from provider to health plan, used for claims adjudication)	ANSI X12-275 (not finalized at the time of publication) and HL7 CDA
Premium payment to health plan*	ANSI X12-820
First report of injury	ANSI X12-148 (not yet issued)

* These are for voluntarily, not mandatory, use by employers, unions, or associations that pay premiums to the health plan on behalf of members.

Source: Compiled by author based on 45 CFR §160.920 and other sources at the Centers for Medicare and Medicaid Services (CMS), accessible at http://www.cms.gov.

cerns. The only identifier to be finalized at the time of this writing is the national provider identifier (NPI).

The NPI is a new, uniform identifier that all providers are required to use beginning in 2008. The NPI is a 10-digit number, and no letters are used. There is no embedded intelligence in the NPI. In other words, nothing in the 10 digits will provide any additional information about the provider other than identifying who or what the provider is. An institutional provider may, under some circumstances, obtain a separate NPI for a "subpart" if the subpart is unique (for example, a division of a hospital system that bills Medicare separately for distinct types of services).

EXHIBIT 7-1

HIPAA Standardized Code Sets

- *International Classification of Diseases, 9th Edition, Clinical Modification (ICD–9–CM)*, Volumes 1 and 2 for the following conditions:
    (1) Diseases
    (2) Injuries
    (3) Impairments
    (4) Other health problems and their manifestations
    (5) Causes of injury, disease, impairment, or other health problems
- *ICD–9–CM* Volume 3, Procedures, for the following procedures or other actions taken for diseases, injuries, and impairments on hospital inpatients reported by hospitals:
    (1) Prevention
    (2) Diagnosis
    (3) Treatment
    (4) Management
- National Drug Codes (NDC) for drugs and biologics
- Code on Dental Procedures and Nomenclature, as maintained and distributed by the American Dental Association, for dental services
- The combination of Health Care Common Procedure Coding System (HCPCS), as maintained and distributed by the Department of Health and Human Services (DHHS), and *Current Procedural Terminology, Fourth Edition* (CPT-4), as maintained and distributed by the American Medical Association (AMA) for physician services and other health care services. These services include, but are not limited to, the following:
    (1) Physician services
    (2) Physical and occupational therapy services
    (3) Radiologic procedures
    (4) Clinical laboratory tests
    (5) Other medical diagnostic procedures
    (6) Hearing and vision services
    (7) Transportation services including ambulance
    (8) Orthotic and prosthetic devices
    (9) Durable medical equipment

Source: Compiled by author based on 45 CFR §160.1002 and other sources at the Centers for Medicare and Medicaid Services (CMS) within the DHHS, accessible at http://www.cms.gov

The NPI replaces all other forms of provider identifiers, such as the Medicare universal provider identification numbers (UPIN), Blue Cross and Blue Shield numbers, health plan provider numbers, TRICARE (a military program beyond the scope of this book) numbers, Medicaid numbers, and so forth. The only provider numbers that are not affected are the taxpayer identifying number and the Drug Enforcement Administration (DEA) number for providers who prescribe or administer prescription drugs. The National Employer Identification Number (EIN) is not affected either, to the extent that a provider is also an employer. The NPI is unique and never-ending in that once assigned a NPI, the provider will use that identifier for all transactions regardless of location, plan type, or anything else.

Privacy

The privacy provisions of HIPAA are highly complex. State provisions are allowed to be stricter than those of HIPAA but not less strict. Under HIPAA, privacy around health information is addressed in several ways that are briefly described as follows.

Protected health information. Central to the privacy and security regulations is the concept of Protected Health Information (PHI). Only information that falls within the definition of PHI is subject to the regulations, and any other information is outside the regulatory scope of HIPAA. Although the privacy and security provisions of HIPAA are separate, they are inextricably linked because of this.

PHI is individually identifiable health information that is transmitted or maintained in electronic media or in any other form or medium. In other words, all electronic, paper, and oral information is covered. Health information is all information that is created or received by a covered entity and that relates to the past, present, or future physical or mental health or condition of an individual; the provision of health care to an individual; or the past, present, or future payment for the provision of health care to an individual. Information is "individually identifiable" either if it identifies the individual, such as by name, or if there is a reasonable basis to believe that the information can be used to identify the individual, such as an address or social security number. Protected health information is intended to be extremely broad and cover most of the information received by an MCO with respect to a health benefits contract.

Consumer control over health information. Patients have the right to understand and control how their health information is used. In particular, the following rules apply under HIPAA:

- Patients should be educated about privacy protections.
- Patients should have access to their medical records.
- Patient consent is required before information is released.
- Patient consent must be voluntary, not coerced.
- Patients should have recourse if their privacy protections are violated.

Limits on medical record use and release. With few exceptions, PHI can be used for health care purposes only. In addition, in any circumstance, only the minimum necessary information should be disclosed (this rule does not apply to the transfer of medical records for the purpose of medical treatment, though). Further, routine disclosures require patient consent, and nonroutine disclosures require patient authorization. The main exception to the requirement that PHI be used only for health care purposes are some defined and limited marketing, fund-raising, and outreach activities by provider organizations; an individual may also choose to "opt out" of any such use.

Examples of routine use of PHI that would apply to all covered entities are the use of it for payment, treatment, and health care operations. For example, a hospital must use PHI to both provide care and to bill an MCO for that care, and an MCO must have enough information to accurately process the claim. Other examples of routine use of PHI by an MCO would be utilization review, disease management, and quality management as described in Chapter 4.

A covered entity must disclose PHI to the individual to whom it is about (or to that person's representative under certain circumstances). A covered entity must also disclose PHI to law enforcement agencies and regulatory bodies under certain conditions. Finally, a covered entity may disclose PHI to a business associate when necessary to conduct routine functions (for example, an MCO may use another company to process its enrollment forms), but the covered entity must have signed assurances that the business associate will comply with all privacy requirements.

Administrative requirements. The HIPAA privacy provisions also have administrative requirements that MCOs must follow. The first of these is that an MCO must provide a notice to its members containing specified information about how PHI will be used and what the member's rights are. An MCO must establish policies and procedures addressing all the privacy requirements and must designate a privacy official who is responsible for the development and implementation of those policies and procedures. An MCO must train its workforce about the HIPAA requirements and take appropriate action if an employee does not comply. The

MCO must also maintain all written records, such as its policies and procedures and all written communications made to members, for 6 years from the date of the document's creation.

Finally, an MCO must establish a process for receiving complaints about potential HIPAA violations and must make efforts to reduce any harmful effects of a known HIPAA violation. An MCO may not retaliate against a member for exercising his or her rights or any other individual for opposing an action that the individual in good faith believes violates the privacy rules, for filing a complaint, or for assisting in an investigation or proceeding relating to a HIPAA violation.

Security Standards Applicable to Electronic Protected Health Information

Even though the HIPAA privacy provisions generally require covered entities to ensure the confidentiality of PHI by appropriately securing it, the HIPAA security rules require additional measures for *electronic* PHI. Electronic PHI is PHI that is transmitted or maintained in electronic media, which includes hard drives and computer disks, Internet, and e-mail. Facsimile transmission, telephone, and paper PHI are not considered electronic PHI (though are still subject to the general privacy requirements as discussed).

The security rules specify 18 different standards for complying with these general principles, and each standard has many additional specifications. The 18 highly complex security requirements are:

1. Security Management Process: Implement policies and procedures to prevent, detect, contain, and correct security violations.
2. Assigned Security Responsibility: Identify the security official who is responsible for development and implementation of the covered entity's security policies and procedures.
3. Workforce Security: Implement policies and procedures to ensure that all members of the covered entity's workforce have access as appropriate to electronic PHI and to prevent those members of the workforce who do not have access from obtaining access.
4. Information Access Management: Implement policies and procedures for authorizing access to electronic PHI.
5. Security Awareness and Training: Implement a security awareness and training program for all workforce members.
6. Security Incident Procedures: Implement policies and procedures to address security incidents. The required specification includes identifying and

responding to suspected or known security incidents, mitigating the harmful effects of an incident, and documenting incidents and their outcomes.

7. Contingency Plan: Establish, and implement if needed, policies and procedures for responding to an emergency or other occurrence, such as a fire or natural disaster, that damages systems containing electronic PHI.

8. Evaluation: Perform periodic evaluation of the procedures, in light of environmental or operational changes, to establish that the covered entity complies with the security standards.

9. Business Associate Contracts: Obtain satisfactory written assurance from any business associate that creates, maintains, or receives electronic PHI that it will implement safeguards of electronic PHI similar to that required of the covered entity.

10. Facility Access Controls: Implement policies and procedures to limit physical access to electronic PHI systems and the facilities in which they are housed.

11. Workstation Use: Implement policies and procedures that specify the functions to be performed, the manner in which those functions are to be performed, and the physical attributes of the surroundings of a specific workstation that can access electronic PHI.

12. Workstation Security: Implement physical safeguards for all workstations that access electronic PHI to restrict access to authorized users.

13. Device and Media Controls: Implement policies and procedures that govern a facility's receipt and removal of hardware and electronic media that contain electronic PHI.

14. Access Control: Implement technical policies and procedures for systems that maintain electronic PHI to allow access only to those individuals or software programs that have been granted access rights.

15. Audit Controls: Implement hardware, software, and/or procedural mechanisms that record and examine activity in information systems that contain electronic PHI.

16. Integrity: Implement policies and procedures to protect electronic PHI from improper alteration or destruction.

17. Person or Identity Authentication: Implement procedures to verify that a person or entity seeking access to electronic PHI is the one claimed.

18. Transmission Security: Implement technical security measures to guard against unauthorized access to electronic PHI that is being transmitted over an electronic communications network.

THE EMPLOYEE RETIREMENT INCOME SECURITY ACT

ERISA has had a direct impact on all health benefits plans and MCOs, especially self-funded plans. As discussed in Chapter 2, an employer has the option of assuming the risk for the medical costs associated with a health benefits plan rather than buying insurance to cover the risk. In a very real sense, a self-insured employer is acting as its own insurance company (within limits). It is rare for a self-insured employer to administer its health plan, however. The more likely strategy is for it to contract with an insurance company or MCO to administer the plan. However, any benefits plan that is self-funded, regardless of how it is administered, falls under the ERISA preemption. As noted earlier in the chapter, this preemption means that a self-funded benefits plan, regardless of how it is administered, is generally not subject to state insurance laws, regulations, or premium taxes. The degree of oversight and regulation is not comparable, however. Although ERISA covers many administrative issues, it addresses health issues in only a very limited degree when compared with state insurance departments.

General Provisions

Even though it does not actually concern the business of insurance, ERISA does apply to aspects of employee benefits in general, including those in insured plans. Regarding these aspects, individual states are allowed to have requirements that are stricter, but not less strict, than those found in ERISA. One of these requirements concerns documentation (e.g., the requirement that a health benefits plan provide consumers with an intelligible description of the plan), and some of them cover the filing of information with the U.S. Department of Labor and the Internal Revenue Service. The most important exception to the divide between federal and state requirements under ERISA, however, involves appeal and grievance rights, which are discussed in the next section.

Under ERISA and except as noted, self-insured employers are not subject to any state laws regarding benefits or premiums or to any other oversight. Indeed, under the act, benefits and costs are hardly regulated at all. What little regulation exists addresses items such as:

- Exclusions for preexisting conditions
- Waiting periods for coverage
- COBRA benefits extension requirements

- HIPAA requirements
- Coverage of children (including adopted children and coverage of children through court order in divorce)
- Pediatric vaccinations
- Coverage for mental health services, maternity care, and mastectomies

However, ERISA preemption is not all-encompassing. For example, state AWP laws as discussed earlier in the chapter are not pre-empted by ERISA. Other laws, such as a surcharge on hospitals, which affects providers and therefore indirectly affects self-funded plans, are also not preempted by ERISA. Finally, ERISA has extensive requirements that must be met regarding the concept of "fiduciary responsibility," which refers to how the plan must provide its benefits responsibly.

Grievances and Appeals

All MCOs are required to have a formal grievance and appeals process, as discussed in Chapter 5. ERISA addresses the appeals process directly, and as noted earlier, the model act used by many states has been revised over the years to more closely align with the federal process described under ERISA. A state may have stricter appeals requirements than are found in ERISA, though those would only apply to insured business, whereas ERISA applies to all. The minimum requirements under ERISA for the formal procedure include the following:

- *Timeliness of response.* ERISA requires urgent care claims to be reviewed in 72 hours or less, whereas some states require 24 hours. ERISA and many states require resolution within 90 days for nonurgent appeals, with an additional 60 days' time for resolution of an appeal of the initial decision. Additional time may be allowed under certain circumstances, such as to accommodate the need for additional information.
- *Who will review the grievance or appeal.* The use of external review bodies is required by many states, primarily for external review of medical necessity decisions. ERISA is slightly less specific, requiring review by an individual or body not involved in the initial decision and requiring that review of any determination based on medical judgment must be conducted in consultation with a health care professional who is independent of the health care professional involved in the initial determination.
- *Limitations on how long a member has to file a grievance or appeal.* ERISA and many state laws require that a member file an appeal to the initial decision

within 180 days of that decision, or else he or she may lose the right under the plan's grievance procedure to file.

- *What recourse a member has.* There are considerable differences in the availability of further recourse to adverse decisions once the grievance and appeals process is exhausted. These differences are based on whether the benefits plan is insured, self-funded, or part of a governmental plan, but ERISA specifically does not provide a right to a trial by jury. ERISA does not preempt state laws requiring additional review options, such as a second review of a decision based on medical judgment.

ACCREDITATION OF MANAGED CARE ORGANIZATIONS

Accreditation is a form of oversight in which an outside organization reviews an MCO and determines if it meets certain criteria. If it meets those criteria (discussed next), it is considered accredited. The difference between accreditation and oversight by a government agency (e.g., a state insurance department) is that the accreditation is completely voluntary, and accrediting organizations are independent, private nonprofit entities. In essence, accreditation is a "seal of approval," and as such, it is relied on by many employers, consumers, and even government agencies.

Accreditation agencies commonly look at an MCO's quality management program and its impact on operations, at utilization management and how it is carried out, at the MCO's treatment of members or consumers, and so forth. The criteria subject to review vary depending on the type of MCO and the accreditation agency performing the review. Next is a brief discussion of the commonly used accreditation agencies in managed care, followed by a description of the Healthcare Effectiveness Data and Information Set (HEDIS) and some of the measures contained in it.

Accreditation Organizations

Three organizations have developed managed care oversight programs of note. They approach their oversight role from different perspectives and specialize in different sectors of the market. The three main accreditation organizations are the National Committee for Quality Assurance (NCQA), URAC (formerly called the Utilization Review Accreditation Commission, but it now uses only the initials), and the Accreditation Association for Ambulatory Health Care (AAAHC, also known as the Accreditation Association). Although each offers related accreditation or certification programs for various types of MCOs, there are some differences that will be briefly discussed. In addition, NCQA has had a special impact on performance measurement in the world of managed care through its development of HEDIS, which is used by roughly 90 percent of all MCOs.

The Joint Commission on Accreditation of Healthcare Organizations (Joint Commission), the dominant organization for facility-based accreditation and certification, discontinued its network accreditation program (for MCOs as well as integrated delivery systems) effective January 1, 2006. However, the Joint Commission provides support services and oversight to organizations accredited under this program through the end of each organization's respective accreditation award period.

All three accrediting organizations offer differing levels of accreditation, depending on how completely the MCO meets or does not meet accreditation standards. Finally, accreditation by any of these three may also be deemed as meeting requirements by Medicare to offer a Medicare Advantage managed care plan (see Chapter 6).

NCQA

For NCQA, the major emphasis is on improving the quality of health care by measuring results and providing the market—consumers and employers—with information that will allow for direct comparisons between the organizations on the basis of quality. For NCQA, quality, effectiveness of care, and member satisfaction performance make up a full 40 percent of accreditation score. Using the objective measures found in HEDIS, NCQA puts emphasis on those mechanisms that the organization has established for continuous improvement in quality. Historically, NCQA focused on evaluating HMO and POS plans, but its agenda has expanded considerably in recent years and now includes behavioral health care organizations, PPOs, credentialing verification organizations (CVOs; see Chapter 3), provider groups and other health care entities.

URAC

URAC was formed in 1990 with the backing of a broad range of consumers, employers, regulators, providers, and industry representatives to provide an efficient and effective method for evaluating utilization review (UR) processes. The organization has since branched out beyond UR oversight and into the evaluation of health plans and PPOs, CVOs, disease management programs, health Web sites, and other health care entities. The stated mission of URAC is "to promote continuous improvement in the quality and efficiency of health care management through processes of accreditation and education." Originally, URAC was incorporated under the name Utilization Review Accreditation Commission. However, that name was shortened to just the acronym URAC in 1996 when URAC began accrediting other types of organizations, such as health plans and PPOs. In addition, URAC sometimes uses a second corporate name, or DBA, which is the American Accreditation HealthCare Commission, Inc.

AAAHC

The AAAHC was formed in 1979 to assist ambulatory health care organizations improve the quality of care provided to patients. The AAAHC accredits more than 2,700 health care organizations, including endoscopy centers, ambulatory surgery centers, office-based surgery centers, student health centers, and large medical and dental group practices. The AAAHC also surveys and accredits managed care organizations and independent physician associations (IPAs; see Chapters 2 and 3). The organization's managed care standards are developed with active industry input and include the evaluation of enrollee communications systems; enrollee complaint and grievance resolution systems; utilization management, including enrollee appeal procedures; quality management and improvement; and provider credentialing and recredentialing systems.

Accreditation by Type of MCO

HMOs have been subjected to external accreditation review more than other types of MCOs. In fact, over 70 percent of HMOs have undergone review. The accreditation process for HMOs is extensive. It looks at quality management, utilization management, wellness and prevention, the treatment of specific diseases and outcomes achieved, provider network composition and access, provider credentialing, financial performance, customer service and member satisfaction, grievance and appeal procedures, and other measures.

PPOs have not undergone accreditation review as commonly as HMOs have, but that is changing. The accreditation process looks at many of the same topics that the process for HMOs does (with some exceptions), including specific diseases. The process tends to be less detailed, which is consistent with the less intensive management-of-care provision characteristic of PPOs, but it is rapidly becoming more sophisticated.

The following additional types of managed care entities and some specific offerings are also the focus of accreditation standards by these organizations:

- Freestanding utilization review organizations
- Disease management programs
- Managed behavioral health care programs
- CVOs
- Physician organizations (e.g., medical groups or IPAs) that perform substantial managed care functions
- Pharmacy benefit management programs
- Physician recognition programs (e.g., meeting certain standards for diabetes care)
- Health Web sites

HEDIS

HEDIS has become an industry standard for reporting data to employers and some government agencies. By specifying not only what to measure but also how to measure it, HEDIS allows true "apples-to-apples" comparisons between health plans. Every year, dozens of national news magazines, local newspapers, employers, and others use HEDIS data to generate health plan "report cards" during open enrollment. All HEDIS data are independently audited and verified. HEDIS, which was developed and is continually refined by NCQA, currently consists of about 60 measures, not including the modified Consumer Assessment of Healthcare Providers and Systems (CAHPS) survey, discussed in the next section, which includes dozens of individual questions. The HEDIS measures fall into six broad categories.

Effectiveness of Care

Measures in this category underlie such oft-reported statistics as childhood immunization rates; cancer screening; appropriate use of antibiotics; management of behavioral health conditions; and common chronic illnesses, including asthma, coronary artery disease, diabetes, and chronic obstructive pulmonary disease (COPD). These and other measures seek to establish whether the health plan is responding to the needs of those who are ill ("Does the health plan make me better when I am sick?") and also to the needs of those who are well ("Does the health plan help me stay healthy when I am well?").

Access/Availability of Care

Measures in this category assess whether care is available to members in a timely manner when they need it and where they need it. Among others, important measures in this category include adults' access to preventive health care, children and adolescents' access to primary care, and women's access to prenatal and post-partum care.

Satisfaction with the Experience

These measures from the CAHPS Health Plan Adult and Child Surveys provide important information about whether a health plan is able to satisfy the diverse needs of its members. Two different surveys—one for adults, the other related to parents' impressions of the care their children receive—include numerous questions related to many key consumer issues, including getting needed care, getting care quickly, how well doctors communicate, helpfulness of office staff, customer service, claims processing, and overall rating of health plan.

Health Plan Stability

These measures—practitioner turnover, years in business, and total membership—provide information about the soundness and dependability of a health plan.

Use of Services

How a health plan uses its resources is a signal of how competently care is managed. Measures in this category permit members and other users to understand patterns of service utilization across different health plans. Measures look at important areas such as the frequency of ongoing prenatal care, well-child and adolescent visits, frequency of selected procedures, inpatient utilization, maternity care length of stay, and several indicators of mental health utilization.

Health Plan Descriptive Information

Although not technically performance measures, HEDIS includes several general questions about aspects of a health plan that employers and consumers have found useful when selecting among plans. These include indicators such as board certification of network physicians, enrollment by product line and state, and racial and ethnic diversity of membership.

The full 2008 HEDIS measure set is listed in Table 7–2.

Table 7–2 2008 HEDIS Measures

EFFECTIVENESS OF CARE

Prevention and Screening
- Childhood Immunization
- Lead Screening in Children
- Breast Cancer Screening
- Cervical Cancer Screening
- Colorectal Cancer Screening
- Chlamydia Screening
- Glaucoma Screening

Respiratory Conditions
- Appropriate Testing for Children with Pharyngitis
- Appropriate Treatment for Children with Upper Respiratory Infection
- Avoidance of Antibiotic Treatment in Adults with Acute Bronchitis
- Use of Spirometry Testing COPD
- Pharmacotherapy Management of COPD Exacerbation
- Use of Appropriate Medications for People with Asthma

Cardiovascular
- Cholesterol Management
- Controlling High Blood Pressure
- Persistence of Beta-Blocker Treatment after a Heart Attack

Diabetes
- Comprehensive Diabetes Care

Musculoskeletal
- Disease Modifying Antirheumatic Drug Therapy for Rheumatoid Arthritis
- Osteoporosis Management in Women
- Imaging Studies for Low Back Pain

Behavior Health
- Antidepressant Medication Management
- Follow-up Care for Children Prescribed ADHD Medication
- Follow-up after Hospitalization for Mental Illness

(continues)

Table 7–2 2008 HEDIS Measures *(continued)*

Medication Management

- Annual Monitoring for Patients on Persistent Medications
- Potentially Harmful Drug-Disease Interactions in the Elderly
- Use of High Risk Medications in the Elderly

Measures Collected through Medicare Health Outcomes Survey

- Medicare Health Outcomes Survey
- Fall Risk Management
- Management of Urinary Incontinence in Older Adults
- Osteoporosis Testing in Older Women
- Physical Activity in Older Adults

Measures Collected through CAHPS Health Plan Survey

- Flu Shots, Ages 50–64
- Flu Shots, Older Adults
- Medical Assistance with Smoking Cessation
- Pneumonia Vaccination Status for Older Adults

Access and Availability

- Adults' Access to Preventive/Ambulatory Services
- Children and Adolescents' Access to PCPs
- Annual Dental Visit
- Initiation and Engagement of Alcohol and Other Drug Dependence Treatment
- Prenatal and Postpartum Care
- Call Abandonment
- Call Answer Timeliness

Satisfaction with the Experience of Care

- CAHPS Health Plan Survey 4.0H, Adult Version
- CAHPS Health Plan Survey 3.0H, Child Version
- Children with Chronic Conditions

Use of Services

- Frequency of Ongoing Prenatal Care
- Well-child Visits/15 months
- Well-child Visits/3–6 years
- Adolescent Well-care Visits
- Frequency of Selected Procedures
- Ambulatory Care
- Inpatient Utilization–General Hospital/Acute Care

(continues)

Table 7–2 2008 HEDIS Measures *(continued)*

- Inpatient Utilization–Nonacute Care
- Identification of Alcohol and Other Drug Services
- Mental Health Utilization
- Antibiotic Utilization
- Outpatient Drug Utilization

Cost of Care

- Relative Resource Use for People with Diabetes
- Relative Resource Use for People with Asthma
- Relative Resource Use for People with Acute Low Back Pain
- Relative Resource Use for People with Cardiovascular Conditions
- Relative Resource Use for People with Uncomplicated Hypertension
- Relative Resource Use for People with COPD

Health Plan Descriptive Information

- Board Certification
- Enrollment by Product Line
- Enrollment by State
- Language Diversity of Membership
- Race/Ethnicity Diversity of Membership
- Weeks of Pregnancy at Time of Enrollment

Health Plan Stability

- Years in Business/Total Membership

Source: NCQA, 2008. Used with permission.

Consumer Assessment of Healthcare Providers and Systems

CAHPS is a multiyear initiative of the Agency for Healthcare Research and Quality (AHRQ) to support the assessment of consumers' experiences with health care. Initially, CAHPS focused only on managed care health plans, but has since expanded its reach. The goals of the CAHPS program are twofold:

- Develop standardized patient questionnaires that can be used to compare results across sponsors and over time

- Generate tools and resources that sponsors can use to produce understandable and usable comparative information for both consumers and health care providers[2]

The first CAHPS survey was developed in 1995 and focused exclusively on Medicare, and then Medicaid HMOs. Primarily concerned with consumers' experiences, it looked at numerous member satisfaction and access-to-care issues. Since then, the health plan version of CAHPS has continued to evolve and become more sophisticated, and it is no longer confined to Medicare and Medicaid plans.

CAHPS for Health Plans asks questions about access to care, communications, and overall satisfaction; how well a consumer feels a health plan carries out its administrative functions; and a number of questions about health status and chronic medical conditions. Specialized versions of CAHPS for Health Plans are used for behavioral health and for children with chronic conditions. NCQA requires that health plans seeking accreditation use a modified version of CAHPS.

The CAHPS Hospital Survey, sometimes known as Hospital CAHPS (H-CAHPS), is a newly developed standardized survey of adult inpatients with hospital care and services. First used in 2006, results will be made public beginning in 2008. This consumer survey asks questions regarding communications between patients and their doctors, nurses, and hospital staff, as well as questions about communications about medications. Additional questions are asked about pain management, general responsiveness and satisfaction, the hospital environment, and around the patient's discharge experience. A specialized version is used for hemodialysis, and a nursing home version is under development.

A version of CAHPS that will focus on clinicians and medical groups is under development. It will look at ambulatory care provided by clinicians in three broad categories: adult primary care, adult specialty care, and child primary care. Similar to the other surveys, it will ask questions about communications, access to care, and how satisfied the consumer is.

CONCLUSION

The managed care industry is heavily regulated and carefully scrutinized. MCOs, no matter what types of benefits plans they are selling and administering, are subject to federal and state laws and regulations. In addition, private nonprofit accreditation

---

[2] https://www.cahps.ahrq.gov/default.asp. Accessed June 13, 2008.

agencies are increasingly reviewing the operations of MCOs to assure consumers, employers, and government agencies that they are meeting quality and performance criteria. Finally, information collected through these various channels is increasingly being made available to consumers.

Portions of this chapter were adapted from D. Horoschak and S. Silva, "State Regulation of Managed Care"; L. Riley and P. Kongstvedt, "HIPAA"; J. Saue and G. Dooge, "ERISA"; and M. O'Kane, "Accreditation and Performance Measurement Programs for Managed Care Organizations" in *The Essentials of Managed Health Care,* 5th edition, ed. P. R. Kongstvedt (Sudbury, MA: Jones & Bartlett Publishers, 2007).

Glossary of Terms and Acronyms*

Access fee—A fee charged by an MCO for access to its provider network, including its reimbursement terms, by an employer or another MCO. See also Rental PPO.

Accrual—The amount of money that is set aside to cover expenses. The accrual is the plan's best estimate of what those expenses are and (for medical expenses) is based on a combination of data from the authorization system, the claims system, the lag studies, and the plan's prior history.

ACG—Ambulatory care group, recently renamed Ambulatory Clinical Group. ACGs are a method of categorizing outpatient episodes. There are 51 mutually exclusive ACGs, which are based on resource use over time and modified by principal diagnosis, age and sex. Also see APG and APC.

---

*These are working definitions of common terms and acronyms in the managed health care industry and related health care sectors. In an industry this dynamic, it is not possible to list every term or acronym in use because new ones come into use faster than any publication can keep up with. Other terms will become obsolete or fall out of use while this book is still in print (this is especially so for government agencies and programs). Some definitions in this glossary may also be disputed by others in the industry; the author is open to receiving communication from any such nitpickers. The glossary is an abridged version of the one found in *The Essentials of Managed Health Care*, 5th edition, ed. P. R. Kongstvedt (Sudbury, MA: Jones & Bartlett Publishers), 2007.

ACR—Adjusted community rate. Used in the past by Medicare managed care plans. It is being phased out and replaced with an acuity-based methodology.

ACS contract—See ASO.

Adjudication—The management and processing of claims by an MCO or health insurance company.

Admitted asset—A financial asset of a health plan that can be converted to cash on short notice. See also Nonadmitted asset, Net worth, and Risk-based capital.

Adverse selection—The problem of attracting members who are sicker than the general population (specifically, members who are sicker than was anticipated when the budget for medical costs was developed).

AHIP—America's Health Insurance Plans. The primary trade organization of managed care organizations. Its areas of focus include legislative and lobbying efforts, education, certification of training in managed health care operations, and representation of the health insurance industry to the public. Initially there were three groups: the Group Health Association of America (GHAA), the American Managed Care and Review Association (AMCRA), and the Health Insurance Association of America (HIAA). These predecessor organizations represented different types of health plan constituencies. GHAA and AMCRA merged to form the American Association of Health Plans (AAHP), which in turn merged with HIAA to form AHIP.

AHP—See Association health plan.

AHRQ—The Agency for Healthcare Research and Quality. A federal agency charged with addressing a wide array of quality-related issues and evidence-based standards of care. An excellent resource for the most current thinking on these topics.

Allowed charge—The maximum charge that an MCO or other payer (such as Medicare or Medicaid) will pay for a specific service, even if the amount billed is greater than the allowed charge. This does not mean that it will be paid, however; cost sharing by the member or beneficiary may still apply—a deductible or coinsurance, for example.

ALOS—See LOS.

Ancillary services—Health care services that are ordered by a physician but provided by some other type of provider—for example, diagnostic testing or physician therapy. Does not apply to inpatient care, ambulatory procedures, or pharmacy.

Annual limit—The maximum amount of coverage that a health plan will provide in a year. This may apply to either the aggregate of all costs in a year (e.g., coverage stops when costs exceed $1 million in a year), or it may apply to a specific service (e.g., no more than 20 behavioral health visits are covered in a year). Does not carry over into the next year. Some HMOs do not have annual limits on charges in the aggregate.

ANSI—The American National Standards Institute. ANSI develops and maintains standards for electronic data interchange. HIPAA mandates the use of ANSI X 12N standards for electronic transactions in the health care system.

APC—Ambulatory patient classification. This is the method that CMS settled on for implementing PPS reimbursement for ambulatory procedures. Like the other methods, this is a way of clustering many different ambulatory procedure codes into groups for purposes of payment.

APG—Ambulatory patient group. A reimbursement methodology developed by 3M Health Information Systems for the CMS but used by some commercial health plans, whereas CMS uses APCs. APGs provide for a fixed reimbursement to an institution for outpatient procedures or visits and incorporate data regarding the reason for the visit and patient data. APGs prevent unbundling of ancillary services. Also see ACG and APC.

ASO—Administrative services only. A contract between an insurance company and a self-funded plan in which the insurance company performs administrative services only and does not assume any risk. Services usually include claims processing but may include other services such as actuarial analysis, enrollment utilization review, and so forth. Also see ERISA.

ASP—Average sales price. A method developed by CMS to calculate what it will pay for certain drugs, particularly biological or injectable drugs. It is based on the average price that manufacturers sell a drug for, not what is charged by whoever is administering the drug. Reimbursement for giving the drug is usually the ASP plus 6%.

Association health plan—An association made up of smaller businesses that group together for purposes of providing health benefits to employees. This may be done by purchasing group health insurance in which all the businesses in the association participate equally, or it may be done by creating a pool of employees sufficiently large so as to self-insure, thereby avoiding benefits mandates and pre-mium taxes. See also MEWA and MET.

Authorization—In the context of managed care, authorization refers to the need to obtain authorization before certain types of health care services are covered. Most commonly used in "gatekeeper"-type HMOs in which a PCP must authorize a referral to a specialist, or the HMO will not pay for the specialist visit. Sometimes referred to as preauthorization or preauth. Sometimes used synonymously with precertification (see Precertification); although no clear distinction is actually made, by convention, authorization is applied more often to specialty referral services, whereas precertification is applied more often to facility-based services.

AWP—Any willing provider. This is a form of state law that requires an MCO to accept any provider willing to meet the terms and conditions in the MCO's contract, regardless of whether the MCO wants or needs that provider. Con-sidered to be an expensive form of anti–managed care legislation. Not to be confused with . . .

AWP—Average wholesale price. Commonly used in pharmacy contracting, the AWP is generally determined through reference to a common source of information.

Back office—An informal term describing the administrative processes of a health plan—for example, claims processing or contract management.

Balance billing—The practice of a provider billing a patient for all charges not paid for by the insurance plan, even if those charges are above the plan's UCR or are considered medically unnecessary. Managed care plans and service plans generally prohibit providers from balance billing except for allowed copays, coinsurance, and deductibles. Such prohibition against balance billing may even extend to the plan's failure to pay at all (e.g., because of bankruptcy).

BD/K—Bed days per thousand members. See Days per thousand.

BPO—Business process outsourcing. A form of outsourcing to a third party that focuses on one or more administrative processes of an MCO, such as claims or enrollment.

Bridge—See Doughnut hole.

Cafeteria plan—An informal term for a flexible benefits plan (see Flexible ben-efits plan).

CAHPS—Consumer Assessment of Healthcare Providers and Systems. Begun by the federal government for use in Medicare and Medicaid managed care plans, it is now also used by commercial health plans. It is maintained by the AHRQ and required as part of the NCQA accreditation process. Its initial focus was on managed health care plans, but it is being expanded to ambulatory providers, hospitals, and the Medicare prescription drug program.

Call center—See Contact center.

Capitation—A set amount of money received or paid out; it is based on membership rather than on services delivered and usually is expressed in units of PMPM. It may be varied by such factors as age and sex of the enrolled member.

Carve-out—Refers to a set of medical services that are "carved out" of the basic arrangement. In term of plan benefits, it may refer to a set of benefits that are carved out and contracted for separately; for example, mental health/substance abuse services may be separated from basic medical/surgical. It may also refer to carving out a set of services from a basic capitation rate with a provider—for example, capitating for cardiac care, but carving out cardiac surgery and paying case rates for that.

Case management—A method of managing the provision of health care to members with high-cost medical conditions. The goal is to coordinate the care so as to both improve continuity and quality of care and lower costs. This generally is a dedicated function in the utilization management department. The official definition of case management according to the Certification of Insurance Rehabilitation Specialists Commission (CIRSC) is "a collaborative process which assesses, plans, implements, coordinates, monitors, and evaluates the options and services required to meet an individual's health needs, using communication and available resources to promote quality, cost-effective outcomes" and "occurs across a continuum of care, addressing ongoing individual needs" rather than being restricted to a single practice setting. When focused solely on high-cost inpatient cases, it may be referred to as large case management or catastrophic case management.

Case mix—The mix of cases in an inpatient setting, accounting for differences in potential or real cost and outcomes. Case mix adjustment refers to a methodology of using case mix to evaluate performance of a provider or project potential costs.

CDH/CDHP—See Consumer-directed health plan.

Certificate of authority (COA)—The license required by an HMO or MCO that is issued by a state after the HMO meets regulatory requirements. A form of state licensure.

Certificate of coverage—see EOC.

CHAMPUS—Civilian Health and Medical Program of the Uniformed Services. The old term for the federal program providing health care coverage to families of military personnel, military retirees, certain spouses and dependents of such personnel, and certain others. Now called TRICARE. See also TRICARE.

Chargemaster—The list of charges a hospital has for each and every thing it can charge for on a pure FFS basis. Also called a charge master. What a hospital is actually paid by an MCO, Medicare, or Medicaid is rarely even close to what is listed on the chargemaster. In fact, only the uninsured are subject to those charges.

Churning—The practice of a provider seeing a patient more often than is medically necessary, primarily to increase revenue through an increased number of services. Churning may also apply to any performance-based reimbursement system in which there is a heavy emphasis on productivity (in other words, rewarding a provider for seeing a high volume of patients whether through fee for service or through an appraisal system that pays a bonus for productivity) The term is also used to describe Medicaid beneficiaries whose eligibility for coverage frequently changes.

Claims—The term used to describe a bill for services from a health care provider to the organization or person responsible for payment. Claims can be paper or electronic.

Claims clearinghouse—A company that accepts claims or other transactions from providers, formats them into HIPAA-compliant standards, and electronically transmits them to the payer.

Claims repricing—An activity in which a rental PPO (see Rental PPO) receives claims submitted by the participating providers, reprices them using the PPO fee schedule, and then transmits the repriced claim to the MCO or insurance company for final processing.

Closed panel—A managed care plan that contracts with physicians on an exclusive basis for services and does not allow those physicians to see patients for another managed care organization. Examples include staff- and group-model HMOs. It could apply to a large private medical group that contracts with an HMO.

CMS—The Centers for Medicare and Medicaid Services. The federal agency that oversees all aspects of health financing for Medicare and, in conjunction with states, Medicaid. Part of DHHS. Once called HCFA.

CMS-1450—A paper claim form used by hospitals and facilities, standardized by CMS. The older name was UB-92. Does not apply to electronic claims. CMS no longer accepts paper claims, though most commercial health plans do.

CMS-1500—A paper claims form used by professionals to bill for services. Developed for Medicare but also used in the commercial sector. Does not apply to electronic claims. CMS no longer accepts paper claims, though most commercial health plans do.

CMS-Hierarchical Condition Categories system (CMS-HCC)—A system that is based on diagnoses made in inpatient and outpatient settings, as well as physician settings of care, and used to adjust payments to MA plans.

COA—See Certificate of authority.

COB—Coordination of benefits. An agreement that uses language developed by the National Association of Insurance Commissioners and prevents double payment for services when a subscriber has coverage from two or more insurance companies or MCOs.

COBRA—Consolidated Omnibus Reconciliation Act. A portion of this act requires employers to offer the opportunity for terminated employees to purchase continuation of health care coverage under the group's medical plan (also see Conversion).

Code sets—Sets of codes used by providers to bill for services. As a practical matter, it is used when discussing the official codes that must be used for any electronic transaction covered under HIPAA. The code sets at the time of publication are ICD-9-CM, CPT-4, NDC, HCPCS, and the Code on Dental Procedures and Nomenclature. Official code sets change over time.

Coinsurance—A provision in a member's coverage that limits the amount of coverage by the plan to a certain percentage, commonly 80%. Coinsurance may also vary depending on whether a service was received from an in-network versus out-of-network provider—for example, 80% for in-network care, 60% for out-of-network care.

Commercial health insurance—Health insurance or HMO coverage for subscribers who are not covered by virtue of a government program such as Medicare, Medicaid, or SCHIP. May be group or direct-pay.

Commission—The money paid to a sales representative, broker, or other type of sales agent for selling the health plan. May be a flat amount of money or a percentage of the premium.

Community rating—The rating methodology required of MCOs under the laws of many states, and occasionally PPOs and indemnity plans under certain circumstances. When required, it usually applies only to the small-group market.

The MCO must obtain the same amount of money per member for all members in the plan. Community rating may allow for variability by allowing the MCO to factor in differences for age, sex, mix (average contract size), and industry factors; not all factors are necessarily allowed under state laws, however. Such techniques are referred to as community rating by class and adjusted community rating. Also see Experience rating.

Compliance—See Corporate compliance.

CON—Certificate of need. The requirement that a health care organization obtain permission from an oversight agency before making changes. Generally applies only to facilities or facility-based services. Varies on a state-to-state basis.

Concurrent review—Refers to utilization management that takes place during the provision of services. Almost exclusively applied to inpatient hospital stays.

Consumer-directed health plan (CDH/CDHP)—A type of health plan that combines a high-deductible health insurance policy with a pretax fund such as an HRA or an HSA. The HRA or HSA is used to pay for qualified services on a first-dollar basis but it is not large enough to cover the entire deductible, the so-called doughnut hole. CDHPs also provide information such as cost data and decision support tools to consumers to promote greater involvement on the part of the consumer in making health care choices.

Contact center—That place within an MCO that supports inbound inquiries across a broad array of media (though most frequently, inbound telephone calls), blended with outbound contact and outreach transactions.

Contract year—The 12-month period that a contract for services is in force. Not necessarily tied to a calendar year.

Contributory plan—A group health plan in which the employees must contribute a certain amount toward the premium cost, with the employer paying the rest.

Conversion—The conversion of a member covered under a group master contract to coverage under an individual contract. This is offered to subscribers who lose their group coverage (e.g., through job loss, death of a working spouse, and so forth) and who are ineligible for coverage under another group contract. See COBRA and HIPAA.

Copayment—That portion of a claim or medical expense that a member must pay out-of-pocket. Usually a fixed amount, such as $20.

Corporate compliance—The function in a health plan or provider charged with ensuring compliance with federal rules and regulations. There are many compliance areas for Medicare; specific compliance requirements exist for privacy and security under HIPAA, and financial requirements under Sarbanes-Oxley. Regulations for Medicare and HIPAA also require the existence of a corporate compliance officer (CCO).

Corporate Practice of Medicine Act—A state law that bars physicians from providing care as an employee of a corporation. The physician can provide care as an individual, as a member of a medical group or partnership, or through a Foundation. See also Foundation model. Corporate practice acts may exist for other types of professions as well; certified public accountants performing attestation services, for example.

Cost sharing—Any form of coverage in which the member pays some portion of the cost of providing services. Usual forms of cost sharing include deductibles, coinsurance, and copayments.

Cost shifting—When a provider cannot cover the cost of providing services under the reimbursement received, the provider raises the prices to other payors to cover that portion of the cost.

CPT-4—Current Procedural Terminology, 4th edition. A set of five-digit codes that apply to medical services delivered. Frequently used for billing by professionals (also see HCPCS).

Credentialing—The most common use of the term refers to obtaining and reviewing the documentation of professional providers. Such documentation includes licensure, certifications, insurance, evidence of malpractice insurance, malpractice history, and so forth. Generally includes both reviewing information provided by the provider as well as verification that the information is correct and complete. A much less frequent use of the term applies to closed panels and medical groups and refers to obtaining hospital privileges and other privileges to practice medicine.

CSR—Customer service representative. An individual who interfaces directly with members in the member services function of an MCO.

Custodial care—Care provided to an individual, primarily for the basic activities of living. May be medical or nonmedical, but the care is not meant to be curative or as a form of medical treatment and is often lifelong. Rarely covered by any form of group health insurance or HMO.

Customer services—See Member services.

CVO—Credentialing verification organization. This is an independent organization that performs primary verification of a professional provider's credentials. The managed care organization may then rely on that verification rather than subjecting the provider to providing credentials independently. This lowers the cost and "hassle" for credentialing. NCQA (see NCQA) has issued certification standards for CVOs.

Data transparency—Refers to an MCO or governmental agency making data about health care cost and quality available to consumers, usually via the Internet.

Date of service—Refers to the date that medical services were rendered. Usually different from the date a claim is submitted.

DAW—Dispense as written. The instruction from a physician to a pharmacist to dispense a brand-name pharmaceutical rather than a generic substitution.

Days per thousand—A standard unit of measurement of utilization. Refers to an annualized use of the hospital or other institutional care. It is the number of hospital days that are used in a year for each thousand covered lives.

Death spiral—An insurance term that refers to a vicious spiral of high premium rates and adverse selection, generally in a free-choice environment (typically, an insurance company or health plan in an account with multiple other plans, or a plan offering coverage to potential members who have alternative choices, such as through an association). One plan ends up having continually higher premium rates such that the only members who stay with the plan are those whose medical costs are so high (and who cannot change because of provider loyalty or benefits restrictions such as preexisting conditions) that they far exceed any possible premium revenue. Called the death spiral because the losses from underwriting mount faster than the premiums can ever recover, and the account eventually terminates coverage, leaving the carrier in a permanent loss position.

Deductible—That portion of a subscriber's (or member's) health care expenses that must be paid out-of-pocket before any insurance coverage applies, commonly $100–$300. May apply only to the out-of-network portion of a point-of-service plan. May also apply only to one portion of the plan coverage (e.g., there may be a deductible for pharmacy services or hospital care, but not for anything else).

Defined benefit—A term of insurance that refers to an employer (or government agency that provides benefits to employees) providing a benefit that is the same regardless of the cost (though cost-sharing with employees is not a part of the definition of defined benefit). In other words, an employee knows what type(s) of insurance or managed health care plans are offered and what the benefits are under each, and the employer's contribution to the cost of that coverage is a function of how expensive that coverage is. This is the most common form of employee health insurance benefit.

Defined contribution—a term of insurance that refers to an employer designating a fixed amount of money for use in purchasing insurance or for funding a retirement account.

Demand management—Services or support that an MCO provides members to lower the demand for acute care services. Includes self-help tools, nurse advice lines, and preventive services.

Dental Content Committee of the American Dental Association—A DSMO under HIPAA that focuses on coding standards for dental procedures.

Dependent—A member who is covered by virtue of a family relationship with the member who has the health plan coverage. For example, one person has health insurance or an HMO through work, and that individual's spouse and children, the dependents, also have coverage under that contract.

Designated Standards Maintenance Organizations—Organizations designated in HIPAA that are charged with making recommendations to DHHS regarding updates to existing standards and the addition of new standards to the transactions and code sets.

DHHS—The United States Department of Health and Human Services. This is the cabinet-level federal agency that oversees many programs, including CMS, which is responsible for Medicare and Medicaid (in conjunction with individual states), as well as oversight of HIPAA and other related federal legislation. Also referred to as HHS.

Direct access—See Open access.

Direct contract model—A managed care health plan that contracts directly with private practice physicians in the community rather than through an intermediary such as an IPA or a medical group. A common type of model in open-panel HMOs.

Direct contracting—A term describing a provider or integrated health care delivery system contracting directly with employers rather than through an insurance company or managed care organization. A superficially attractive option that occasionally works when the employer is large enough. Not to be confused with direct contract model (see previous entry). Rarely used for long because it is almost always more costly than working through an existing health plan.

Direct-pay subscriber—An individual subscriber to a health plan who is not covered under a group policy but rather pays the health plan directly. May be a commercial member who has passed underwriting screening, or may be a conversion plan holder (see Conversion). Is not used to describe Medicare or Medicaid subscribers by convention; even though such subscribers are enrolled individually, part or all of their premiums are paid via a government agency.

Discharge planning—That part of utilization management that is concerned with arranging for care or medical needs to facilitate discharge from the hospital.

Disease management—The process of intensively managing a particular disease. This differs from large case management in that it goes well beyond a given case in the hospital, or an acute exacerbation of a condition. Disease management encompasses all settings of care and places a heavy emphasis on prevention and maintenance. Similar to case management but more focused on a defined set of diseases.

Disenrollment—The process of termination of coverage. Voluntary termination would include a member quitting because he or she simply wants out. Involuntary termination would include leaving the plan because of changing jobs. A rare and serious form of involuntary disenrollment is when the plan terminates a member's coverage against the member's will. This is usually only allowed (under state and federal laws) for gross offenses such as fraud, abuse, nonpayment of premium or copayments, or a demonstrated inability to comply with recommended treatment plans.

Dispensing fee—The fee paid to a pharmacy for that part of the cost of a prescription that is not the ingredient cost. Usually a flat dollar amount not tied to the cost of the drug.

Distribution channel—An informal term used to describe the various ways that an MCO sells its products—for example, brokers, consultants, employed sales force, electronic sales portals, and so forth.

DME—Durable medical equipment. Medical equipment that is not disposable (i.e., is used repeatedly) and is only related to care for a medical condition. Examples would include wheelchairs, home hospital beds, and so forth. An area of increasing expense, particularly in conjunction with case management.

DOL—U.S. Department of Labor. Regulates coverage offered to employees when employers retain the insurance risk (i.e., self-funding pursuant to ERISA), either on a stand-alone basis or through a multiple employer welfare arrangement.

Doughnut hole—The term applied to the difference between when first dollar coverage stops and insurance then begins. Also referred to as a bridge. May be applied in a CDHP plan to the gap between the HRA or HSA, and when the high-deductible insurance plan starts to cover costs. Also exists in the basic Medicare Part D drug benefit passed under the MMA, at least at the time of publication. A term that may not necessarily have great persistency.

DRG—Diagnosis-related groups. A statistical system of classifying any inpatient stay into groups for purposes of payment. DRGs may be primary or secondary, and an outlier classification also exists. This is the form of reimbursement that the CMS used to pay hospitals for Medicare recipients. Also used by a few states for all payers and by many private health plans for contracting purposes. DRGs were replaced by MS-DRGs during 2008–2009. See also MS-DRG.

DSM-IV—*Diagnostic and Statistical Manual of Mental Disorders*, 4th edition. The manual used to provide a diagnostic coding system for mental and substance abuse disorders. Far different from ICD-9-CM (see ICD-9-CM).

DSMO—See Designated Standards Maintenance Organization.

Dual eligibles—Individuals who are entitled to both Medicare and Medicaid coverage.

DUR—Drug utilization review.

EAP—Employee assistance program. A program that a company puts into effect for its employees to provide them with help in dealing with personal problems such as alcohol or drug abuse, mental health or stress issues, and so forth.

ED—Emergency Department. That location or department in a hospital or other institutional facility that is focused on caring for acutely ill or injured patients. In earlier times, this was often a room or set of rooms, hence the older designation emergency room, or ER. These days, at least in busy urban and suburban hospitals, volume is high and physicians are specially trained and certified in emergency care, and it has grown to be an entire department.

EDI—Electronic data interchange. A term that refers to the exchange of data through electronic means rather than by using paper or the telephone. Prior to the rise of the Internet, EDI was applied primarily to direct electronic communications via proprietary means. EDI now encompasses electronic data exchange via both proprietary channels and the Internet.

Effective date—The day that health plan coverage goes into effect or is modified.

EFT—electronic funds transfer. Getting paid by electronic transfer of funds directly to one's bank instead of receiving a paper check.

EHR—See electronic health record.

Electronic health record—A more expansive type of electronic record encompassing more than the care provided by a single provider or entity to a single patient.

Electronic medical record—An electronic version of the type of health record that a physician or a hospital keeps on a single patient.

Eligibility—When an individual is eligible for coverage under a plan. Also used to determine when an individual is no longer eligible for coverage (e.g., a dependent child reaches a certain age and is no longer eligible for coverage under his or her parent's health plan).

EMR—See electronic medical record.

EMTALA—The Emergency Medical Treatment and Active Labor Act. 1986. 42, USC 1395 dd (1986) Pub. L. No. 99-272, 9121. "Anti-dumping" legislation dictates that all patients presenting to any hospital emergency department must have a medical screening exam performed by qualified personnel, usually the emergency physician. The medical screening exam cannot be delayed for insurance reasons, either to obtain insurance information or to obtain preauthorization for examination.

Encounter—An outpatient or ambulatory visit by a member to a provider. Applies primarily to physician office visits but may encompass other types of encounters as well. In fee-for-service plans, an encounter also generates a claim. In capitated plans, the encounter is still the visit, but no claim is generated.

Enrollee—An individual enrolled in a managed health care plan. Usually applies to the subscriber or person who has the coverage in the first place rather than to his or her dependents, but the term is not always used that precisely.

EOB—Explanation of benefits (statement). A statement mailed to a member or covered insured explaining how and why a claim was or was not paid; the Medicare version is called an EOMB (also see ERISA).

EOC—Evidence of coverage, also known as a certificate of benefits. The EOC is a document that describes the health care benefits covered by the health plan. It provides the member with some form of documentation that he or she in fact does have health insurance, and it describes what that insurance covers and how it works.

EPO—Exclusive provider organization. An EPO is similar to an HMO in that it often uses primary physicians as gatekeepers, often capitates providers, has a limited provider panel, uses an authorization system, and so forth. It is referred to as exclusive because the member must remain within the network to receive benefits. The main difference is that EPOs are generally regulated under insurance statutes rather than HMO regulations. Not allowed in many states that maintain that EPOs are really HMOs. Now uncommon.

ER—Emergency room; see ED.

ERISA—Employee Retirement Income Security Act. One provision of this act allows self-funded plans to avoid paying premium taxes, avoid complying with state-mandated benefits, and generally avoid complying with state laws and regulations regarding insurance, even when insurance companies and managed care plans that stand risk for medical costs must do so. Another provision requires that plans and insurance companies provide an explanation of benefits (EOB) statement to a member or covered insured in the event of a denial of a claim, explaining why the claim was denied and informing the individual of his or her rights of appeal. Numerous other provisions in ERISA are very important for a managed care organization to know.

ESRD—End stage renal disease. No other particular clinical definitions are found in this glossary; this one is included only because Medicare treats beneficiaries with ESRD differently than other types for purposes of enrollment in MA plans.

Ethics in Referrals Act—See Stark regulations.

Evidence of insurability—The form that documents whether an individual is eligible for health plan coverage when the individual does not enroll through an open enrollment period. For example, if an employee wants to change health plans in the middle of a contract year, the new health plan may require evidence of insurability (often both a questionnaire and a medical exam) to ensure that it will not be accepting adverse risk.

Exclusion—As used in managed care and health insurance, exclusions refer to those services or conditions for which there will be no (or very limited) coverage. The most common is an exclusion in an individual direct-pay policy for preexisting conditions, in which there will be no coverage for conditions that existed at the time the policy was issued. There is also usually a time limit for this type of exclusion; for example, after 2 years, coverage will apply. An exclusion may also be a complete one, such as no coverage for experimental or scientifically unproven care.

Experience rating—The method of setting premium rates based on the actual health care costs of a group or groups.

Experimental and investigational treatment—The term used by MCOs and insurance companies to refer to medical care that is not yet proved or that may be the subject of clinical investigation. Most plans will not cover costs for this unless the patient is enrolled in a qualified investigational trial.

Extracontractual benefits—Health care benefits beyond what the member's actual policy covers. These benefits are provided by a plan to reduce utilization. For example, a plan may not provide coverage for a hospital bed at home, but it is more cost effective for the plan to provide such a bed than to keep admitting a member to the hospital.

Favored nations discount—A contractual agreement between a provider and a payer stating that the provider will automatically provide the payer the best discount it provides anyone else. Prohibited in many states.

Fee schedule—May also be referred to as fee maximums or as a fee allowance schedule. A listing of the maximum fee that a health plan will pay for a certain service, based on CPT billing codes.

FEHBP—Federal Employee Health Benefits Program. The program that provides health benefits to federal employees.

FFS—Fee-for-service. A patient sees a provider, and the provider bills the health plan or patient and gets paid based on that bill. In the case of a contracted provider, the maximum payment may be limited to the fee schedule.

Fiscal intermediary—A company that processes the administrative transactions on behalf of Medicare, though the term may also be used by similar types of companies providing services to state Medicaid programs. May be limited to adjudication and payment of claims or may encompass other activities as well.

Flexible benefits plan—A benefits plan at a company that allows an employee to select from different options up to a set amount of money and always includes an FSA. Also called a cafeteria plan or a Section 125 plan.

Flexible spending account (FSA)—A financial account that is part of a Section 125 plan, funded with pretax dollars via payroll deduction by an employer. Funds may be used to reimburse the employee for qualified expenses not covered under insurance. FSAs exist for health care and, separately, for child care services. Unused FSA funds do not roll into following years; they are "use it or lose it," although in some cases, unused FSA funds can roll over into an HSA account.

Formulary—A listing of drugs that a health plan provides coverage for, but almost always at differing levels. For example, drugs considered Tier 1 in the formulary may be covered with a $5 copay, Tier 2 at a $20 copay, and Tier 3 at a $50 copay. May also list drugs that require precertification for coverage or that are subject to other coverage limitations.

Foundation—A not-for-profit form of integrated health care delivery system. The foundation model is usually formed in response to tax laws that affect not-for-profit hospitals or in response to states with laws prohibiting the corporate practice of medicine (see Corporate Practice Acts). The foundation purchases both the tangible and intangible assets of a physician's practice, and the physicians then form a medical group that contracts with the foundation on an exclusive basis for services to patients seen through the foundation.

FPP—Faculty practice plan. A form of group practice organized around a teaching program. It may be a single group encompassing all the physicians providing services to patients at the teaching hospital and clinics, or it may be multiple groups drawn along specialty lines (e.g., psychiatry, cardiology, or surgery).

FSA—See flexible spending account.

FTE—Full-time equivalent. The equivalent of one full-time employee. For example, two part-time employees are 0.5 FTE each, for a total of 1 FTE.

Full professional risk capitation—A loose term used to refer to a physician group or organization receiving capitation for all professional expenses, not just for the services they themselves provide; it does not include capitation for institutional services (see Global capitation). The group is then responsible for subcapitating or otherwise reimbursing other physicians for services to their members.

Gatekeeper—An informal though widely used term that refers to a primary care case management model health plan. In this model, all care from providers other than the primary care physician, except for true emergencies, must be authorized by the primary care physician before care is rendered. This is a predominant feature of most (but not all) HMOs.

Generic drug—A drug that is equivalent to a brand-name drug but usually less expensive. Most managed care organizations that provide drug benefits cover generic drugs, and may require a member to pay a higher copay for a brand-name drug.

Global capitation—The term used when an organization receives capitation for all medical services, including institutional and professional.

Grace period—The amount of time that an MCO or insurance company must allow a group or individual that hasn't paid their premium to make good on the payment before the plan can cancel the policy. If the delinquent company or individual pays up during the grace period, the policy is said to be reinstated, and coverage is considered unbroken.

Group—The members who are covered by virtue of receiving health plan coverage at a single company.

Group health insurance—A commercial health insurance or HMO coverage policy that is sold to an employer to provide coverage to employees. Does not apply to a conversion policy or a direct-pay policy, nor to Medicare or Medicaid plans.

Group model HMO—An HMO that contracts with a medical group for the provision of health care services. The relationship between the HMO and the medical group is generally very close, although there are wide variations in the relative independence of the group from the HMO. A form of closed-panel health plan.

Group practice—The American Medical Association defines group practice as three or more physicians who deliver patient care, make joint use of equipment and personnel, and divide income by a prearranged formula.

Group Practice without Walls (GPWW)—A group practice in which the members of the group come together legally but continue to practice in private offices scattered throughout the service area. Sometimes called a Clinic without Walls (CWW).

HCFA—Health Care Financing Administration. The older term for CMS, no longer used.

HCPCS—Healthcare (previously HCFA) Common Procedural Coding System. A set of codes used by Medicare that describe services and procedures. HCPCS includes CPT codes but also has codes for services not included in CPT, such as DME and ambulance. Although HCPCS is nationally defined, there is provision for local use of certain codes.

HDHP—High-deductible health plan; see high-deductible health insurance.

Health care—You probably think you know what this means, eh? Well, maybe, maybe not. The term is generally used to refer to the services that a health care professional or institution provides you (e.g., services from a physician, at a hospital, from a physical therapist, and so forth); it is this use of the term that is universally used when discussing care management. There is a broader definition, however, that encompasses services from nontraditional providers and, more important, the health care that individuals self-administer (which is actually the majority of health care anyone receives). When individuals use the broad sense of the term "health care," they frequently use "medical care" to refer to what is considered the narrow meaning just noted. Broad or narrow, it's your choice depending on the context.

Health reimbursement account/arrangement (HRA)—A financial account associated with a CDHP and used to pay for first-dollar qualified health care expenses up to a preset limit using pretax funds provided by an employer. Unused HRA funds may roll into the next year, but they do not follow an individual when he or she changes employment. Always associated with a high-deductible health insurance policy. Not to be confused with . . .

Health risk appraisal (HRA)—Instrument designed to elicit or compile information about the health risk of any given individual. Initially these tools were fairly uniform, but they have now become quite specialized and targeted toward particular populations with distinctive risk profiles (e.g., Medicare, Medicaid, underserved, commercial population, and so forth).

Health savings account (HSA)—Created under the MMA, an HSA is a financial account of pretax dollars for current or future qualified medical expenses, retirement, or long-term care premium expenses. Unused funds roll into following years. Funding may come from an employer and/or an individual and do follow an individual when he or she changes employment. Always associated with a qualified high-deductible health insurance policy. Regulated under tax law.

Healthcare Integrity and Protection Data Bank—An electronic data bank established under HIPAA that records information about providers around fraud and abuse, criminal convictions, civil judgments, injunctions, licensure restrictions, and exclusion from participation in any government programs.

HEDIS—Healthcare Effectiveness Data and Information Set. Developed by NCQA with considerable input from the employer community and the managed care community, HEDIS is an ever-evolving set of data reporting standards. HEDIS is designed to provide some standardization in performance reporting for financial, utilization, membership, clinical data, and more. Employers and consumers then can compare performance between plans if the plan reports HEDIS data. The initial focus was on HMOs, but it has become much more varied.

HHS—Health and Human Services; see DHHS.

High-deductible health insurance/high-deductible health plan—Just what it sounds like, a health insurance policy with a very high deductible, such as $1,500 or even $5,000 per year. The deductible for an individual will be different from an aggregate deductible for a family. Also associated with MSAs, HRAs, and HSAs, high-deductible insurance is a mainstay in a typical CDHP.

HIPAA—Health Insurance Portability and Accountability Act. Enacted in 1997, this act creates a rather vaguely worded set of requirements that allow for insurance portability (i.e., the ability to keep your health insurance even if you move or change jobs), guaranteed issue of all health insurance products to small groups (but only if they have met requirements for prior continuous coverage), and mental health parity (i.e., the dollar limits on mental health coverage cannot be less than that for medical coverage; it is silent, however, to the issues of differential visit limitations, differential coinsurance requirements, or restrictions on networks). More important, HIPAA also contains significant provisions regarding "administrative simplification" and standards for privacy and security. Administrative simplification also mandated the use of certain standards for types of electronic transactions (e.g., electronic claims) and code sets. HIPAA also requires the use of a national provider identifier (see NPI) by providers.

HL7—Health Level 7. A DSMO under HIPAA, HL7 focuses on electronic connectivity standards for clinical information.

HMO—Health maintenance organization. The definition of an HMO has changed substantially. Originally, an HMO was defined as a prepaid organization that provided health care to voluntarily enrolled members in return for a preset amount of money on a PMPM basis. With the increase in self-insured business, or with financial arrangements that do not rely on prepayment, that definition is no longer accurate. Now the definition needs to encompass two possibilities: a licensed health plan (licensed as an HMO, that is) that places at least some of the providers at risk for medical expenses, and a health plan that utilizes designated (usually primary care) physicians as gatekeepers (although there are some HMOs that do not). Many in the field have given up and now use the looser term "MCO" because it avoids having to make difficult definitions like this one.

Hold harmless clause—A contractual clause between a provider and an MCO that prohibits the provider from balance billing a member even in the event that the MCO fails to pay the provider (i.e., the provider holds the member harmless).

Hospice—A program or facility dedicated to palliative care at the end of life. May be a combination of a home care program, an outpatient facility, and/or an inpatient facility.

Hospital-based physician—A specialty physician who practices primarily within a hospital or ambulatory surgical center in one of three clinical areas—anesthesia, radiology, pathology—or who is a hospitalist. See also Hospitalist.

Hospitalist—A physician who concentrates solely on hospitalized patients. In an MCO or medical group, this physician may specialize in hospital care, or the duties may be undertaken on a rotating basis. May also be employed by the hospital. This model allows the other physicians to concentrate on outpatient care, whereas the hospitalist focuses on the care of all the plan's or group's patients in the hospital. In large hospitals with very active intensive care units, a specialized type of hospitalist, called an intensivist, focuses only on caring for the critically ill.

HRA—An acronym that stands for either health risk appraisal or health reimbursement account, depending on circumstances. See Health risk appraisal or Health reimbursement account.

HSA—See Health savings account.

IBNR—Incurred but not reported. The amount of money that the plan had better accrue for medical expenses that it knows nothing about yet. These are medical expenses that the authorization system has not captured and for which claims have not yet hit the door.

ICD-9-CM—International Classification of Diseases, 9th revision, clinical modification. The classification of disease by diagnosis codified into 6-digit numbers. It will eventually be replaced by ICD-10, which is approximately 10 times the size of ICD-9.

IDN—See IDS.

IDS—Integrated delivery system, also referred to as an integrated health care delivery system. Another acronym that means the same thing is IDN (integrated delivery network). An IDS is an organized system of health care providers that spans a broad range of health care services. Although there is no clear definition of an IDS, in its full flower, an IDS should be able to access the market on a broad basis, optimize cost and clinical outcomes, accept and manage a full range of financial arrangements to provide a set of defined benefits to a defined population, align financial incentives of the participants (including physicians), and operate under a cohesive management structure. Also see IPA, PHO, MSO, Staff model, and Foundation.

Indemnity insurance—Insurance that "indemnifies" the policy holder from losses. In health insurance, this applies to providing financial coverage for health care costs, with little or no attempt to manage that cost (other than, perhaps, a precertification program); most important, it is not based on a contracted network of providers, unlike a service plan that may otherwise appear the same. Indemnity insurance plans do limit the amount that they will pay for a professional service, however, based on a some form of fee scale; such limits are rarely in place for institutional costs, however. Once common, indemnity plans are quite rare now because of high cost.

Independent review organization—An independent group that an MCO contracts with to provide a secondary external review of coverage denials based on medical reasons. Required in some states, which may also require that a designated IRO be approved by the state's department of insurance.

Individual policy—An individual, single policy, not a group policy, pays the MCO directly.

Informatics—A loosely defined term that refers to using data mining to create usable reports. It is intended to imply a more sophisticated approach to obtaining and using data than is used for routine operations. The term is preferentially used by many MCOs for the function and/or department that analyzes medical data.

Intensivist—A type of hospitalist (physician) who focuses solely on care provided in the intensive (or critical) care unit.

Intermediary—See Fiscal intermediary.

Investigational treatment—See Experimental and investigational treatment.

IPA—Independent practice association. An organization that has a contract with a managed care plan to deliver services in return for a single capitation rate. The IPA in turn contracts with individual providers to provide the services either on a capitation basis or on a fee-for-service basis. The typical IPA encompasses all specialties, but an IPA can be solely for primary care or may be single specialty. An IPA may also be the "PO" part of a PHO.

IRO—See Independent review organization.

IT—Information technology. A blanket term referring to all the computer hardware and software systems that support the operations of a health plan. Virtually all operational functions of a health plan are supported by IT in one way or another.

JCAHO (Joint Commission)—Joint Commission for the Accreditation of Healthcare Organizations. A not-for-profit organization that performs accreditation reviews primarily on hospitals, other institutional facilities, and outpatient facilities. Most managed care plans require any hospital under contract to be accredited by the Joint Commission.

Lapse—To drop coverage. This may refer to an individual who stops paying premium, thereby allowing her or his policy to lapse, subject to a grace period (see Grace period). When used as a ratio, it is the opposite of a persistency ratio (i.e., the percentage of commercially enrolled groups that drop the health plan).

Legend drug—A drug that can only be provided with a prescription from a licensed provider.

Line of business—A health plan (e.g., an HMO, EPO, or PPO) that is set up as a line of business within another, larger organization, usually an insurance company. This legally differentiates it from a freestanding company or a company set up as a subsidiary. It may also refer to a unique product type (e.g., Medicaid) within a health plan.

LOS/ELOS/ALOS—Length of stay/estimated length of stay/average length of stay.

Loss ratio—See Medical loss ratio.

MA local plan—A Medicare Advantage managed care plan that does not provide services throughout an entire region as designated by CMS.

MA MSA—A Medicare Advantage MSA plan (see also MSAs). MSA plans are not network plans in the sense of being able to limit coverage to a network. Enrollees of such plans have the right to expect the plan to cover the cost of care at any provider willing to accept the individual as a patient, consistent with the rules of the plan regarding coverage (e.g., an MSA plan has no coverage before a deductible is met).

MA regional plan—A Medicare Advantage PPO-type plan that provides services throughout an entire region as designated by CMS.

MAC—Maximum allowable charge (or cost). The maximum, although not the minimum, that a vendor may charge for something. This term is often used in pharmacy contracting; a related term, used in conjunction with professional fees, is fee maximum.

Managed behavioral health care organization (MBHO)—A third party that manages the behavioral health services benefits for an MCO. It may also contract directly with an employer. An MBHO may be at financial risk, or it may manage the services under an administrative contract only. A form of clinical outsourcing.

Managed health care—A regrettably nebulous term. At the very least, it is a system of health care delivery that tries to manage the cost of health care, the quality of that health care, and access to that care. Common denominators include a panel of contracted providers that is smaller than the entire universe of available providers, some type of limitations on benefits to subscribers who use noncontracted providers (unless authorized to do so), and some type of authorization or precertification system. Managed health care is actually a spectrum of systems ranging from so-called managed indemnity, through CDHPs, POS plans, PPOs, open-panel HMOs, and closed-panel HMOs. For a better definition, the reader is urged to read this book and formulate his or her own.

Mandated benefits—Benefits that a health plan is required to provide by law. This is generally used to refer to benefits above and beyond routine insurance-type benefits, and it generally applies at the state level (where there is high variability from state to state). Common examples include in-vitro fertilization, defined days of inpatient mental health or substance abuse treatment, and other special-condition treatments. Self-funded plans are exempt from most mandated benefits under ERISA, but even the federal government gets into the act, with a mandatory 2-day length of stay for childbirth, and mental health parity provisions under HIPAA that apply to both insured and self-funded plans.

Mandatory external review—The requirement that an MCO provide a means for a physician or member who appeals a decision about medical coverage to obtain a second opinion from an unbiased external reviewer, a physician in a specialty appropriate for the clinical condition. This process has been mandated in some states and is widely undertaken on a voluntary basis in any event.

Master group contract—The actual contract between a health plan and a group that purchases coverage. The master group contract provides specific terms of coverage, rights, and responsibilities of both parties.

Maximum out-of-pocket cost—The most amount of money a member will ever need to pay for covered services during a contract year. The maximum out-of-pocket includes deductibles and coinsurance. Once this limit is reached, the health plan pays for all services up to the maximum level of coverage. Applies mostly to non-HMO plans such as indemnity plans, CDHPs, PPOs, and POS plans.

MBHO—See Managed behavioral health care organization.

MCO—Managed care organization. A generic term applied to a managed care plan. In the past decade or so, some initially used the term "MCO" to refer to an HMO simply because they thought that there was less negative connotation. However, it now encompasses plans that do not conform exactly to the strict definition of an HMO (although that definition has itself loosened considerably) and may also apply to a PPO, EPO, CDHP, IDS, or even an OWA.

Medical loss ratio—The ratio between the cost to deliver medical care and the amount of money that was taken in by a plan. Insurance companies often have a medical loss ratio of 92% or more; tightly managed HMOs may have medical loss ratios of 75% to 85%, although the overhead (or administrative cost ratio) is concomitantly higher. The medical loss ratio is dependent on the amount of money brought in and the cost of delivering care; thus, if the rates are too low, the ratio may be high, even though the actual cost of delivering care is not really out of line. May also be called the medical expense ratio (MEO).

Medical policy—Policies of a health plan regarding what will be paid for as medical benefits. Routine medical policy is linked to routine claims processing and is automated in the claims system; for example, the plan may only pay 50% of the fee of a second surgeon, or it may not pay for two surgical procedures done during one episode of anesthesia. This also refers to how a plan approaches payment policy for experimental or investigational care, and payment for noncovered services in lieu of more expensive covered services.

Medically necessary—The term used to refer to whether a clinical service or supply (e.g., a drug or a device) is actually necessary to protect or preserve the health of an individual, based on evidence-based medical knowledge or practices. Not always easy to define in any particular circumstance.

Medicare—Social health insurance provided by the federal government for citizens over the age of 65 and some others, such as individuals with end-stage renal disease. Regular Medicare is a FFS type of insurance; Part A covers hospital care, and Part B covers professional services. Medicare now also provides a drug benefit under Part D, passed under the MMA. Traditional FFS Medicare is administered by intermediaries performing on behalf of CMS, whereas Medicare Advantage uses various forms of private health plans.

Medicare Advantage (MA)—Created as part of the MMA, MA replaced and expanded other forms of Medicare managed care. MA plans may be HMOs, PPOs, or PFFS plans; they may also be local or regional. Special Needs Plans (SNPs) were also created to focus on specific types of beneficiaries. MA MSAs are also overseen under MA.

Medicare Modernization Act of 2003 (MMA)—The federal act originally titled the Medicare Prescription Drug Improvement and Modernization Act of 2003. The MMA is the basis for both the Medicare Part D drug benefit and for the variety of MA plans described elsewhere, including MA local, MA regional, and MA PFFS.

Medigap insurance—A form of state-licensed health insurance that covers whatever Medicare does not. Medigap policies are subject to minimum standards under federal law and have been further restricted under the MMA.

Member—An individual covered under a managed care plan. May be either the subscriber or a dependent.

Member months—The total of all months that each member was covered. For example, if a plan had 10,000 members in January and 12,000 members in February, the total member months for the year to date as of March 1 would be 22,000.

Member services—The department, as well as the actual services, that support a member's needs, not including the actual provision of health care. Examples of such member services include resolving problems, managing disputes by members about coverage issues, managing the grievance and appeals processes, and so forth. Member services also function in a proactive manner, reaching out to members with educational programs, self-service capabilities, and the like. Also known as customer services.

Mental Health Parity Act—Passed by Congress in 1996, it requires group health plans that offer mental health coverage benefits to apply the same annual and aggregate lifetime dollar limits to mental health coverage as those applied to coverage of other services. The federal law applies to fully insured and self-insured plans, including state-regulated plans. However, states may enact requirements more stringent than those contained under the federal law.

Messenger model—A type of IDS that simply acts as a messenger between an MCO and the providers participating in the IDS regarding contracting terms. Does not have the power to collectively bargain, thus avoiding antitrust violations.

MET—Multiple employer trust. See MEWA.

MEWA—Multiple employer welfare association. A group of employers who band together for purposes of purchasing group health insurance, often through a self-funded approach to avoid state mandates and insurance regulation. By virtue of ERISA, such entities are regulated little, if at all. Many MEWAs have enabled small employers to obtain cost-effective health coverage, but some MEWAs have not had the financial resources to withstand the risk of medical costs and have failed, leaving the members without insurance or recourse. In some states, MEWAs and METs are no longer legal. See also Association health plan.

MIS—Management information system. An older term for the computer hardware and software that provides the support for managing the plan. See also IT (the more commonly used term).

Mixed model—A managed care plan that mixes two or more types of delivery systems. This has traditionally been used to describe an HMO that has both closed-panel and open-panel delivery systems.

MLP—Midlevel practitioner. Physician's assistants, clinical nurse practitioners, nurse midwives, and the like. Nonphysicians who deliver medical care, generally under the supervision of a physician but for less cost.

MMA—See Medicare Modernization Act.

MSA—Medical savings account. Created as a demonstration under BBA '97 and updated in the MMA, MSAs are specialized savings accounts into which a consumer can put pretax dollars for use in paying medical expenses in lieu of purchasing a comprehensive health insurance or managed care product. MSAs require a catastrophic health insurance policy as a "safety net" to protect against very high costs. They still exist, in both commercial form and for Medicare, but they have been supplanted by CDHPs that are similar in approach but have additional features that make them more attractive to the market.

MS-DRG—Medicare Severity Diagnosis-Related Groups. Implemented by Medicare to replace traditional DRGs. MS-DRGs are not only based on the diagnosis and procedures performed but also take into account other chronic conditions and comorbidities, including major chronic conditions and comorbidities. With the advent of MS-DRGs in 2008–2009, fewer cases will qualify as outliers.

MSO—Management service organization. A form of integrated health delivery system. Sometimes similar to a service bureau (see Service bureau), the MSO often actually purchases certain hard assets of a physician's practice and then provides services to that physician at fair market rates. MSOs are usually formed as a means to contract more effectively with managed care organizations, although their simple creation does not guarantee success.

Mutual company—A type of not-for-profit health insurance company or Blue Cross Blue Shield plan that is legally owned by the policy holders, not the community nor private investors.

NAIC—National Association of Insurance Commissioners.

National Practitioner Data Bank—A data bank established under the federal Health Care Improvement and Quality Act of 1986, it electronically stores information about physician malpractice suits successfully litigated or settled, and disciplinary actions on physicians. This information is accessible to hospitals and health plans under controlled circumstances as part of the credentialing process. Hospitals and health plans must likewise report disciplinary actions to the data bank.

National Quality Forum—A not-for-profit public/private organization created to develop and implement a national strategy for health care quality measurement and reporting. It is a voluntary consensus standards-setting organization addressing quality measurements in such things as pay for performance, electronic health records, patient safety, and so forth.

NCPDP—National Council for Prescription Drug Programs. The NCPDP, which developed and maintains the accepted electronic data interchange standard for pharmacy claims transmission and adjudication, accelerated the adoption of pharmacy e-commerce. This standard permits the submission of pharmacy claims and the adjudication of those claims in a real-time interactive mode. Recognized by ANSI and addressed under HIPAA.

NCQA—National Committee on Quality Assurance. A not-for-profit organization that performs quality-oriented accreditation reviews on HMOs and similar types of managed care plans. NCQA also now accredits CVOs, PPOs, certain types of DM programs, and so forth. NCQA developed and maintains the HEDIS standards.

NDC—National drug code. The national classification system for identifying prescription drugs.

Net worth—For purposes of health insurance and managed care, net worth is what a health plan has in assets that can be readily converted into cash in the event of plan failure, such as unrestricted cash or investments, or other equally liquid and unencumbered assets. States have net worth minimum requirements for licensed health plans that vary with the size of the potential liability. See also Nonadmitted asset and Risk-based capital.

Network-model HMO—A health plan that contracts with multiple physician groups to deliver health care to members. Generally limited to large single- or multispecialty groups. Distinguished from group model plans that contract with a single medical group, IPAs that contract through an intermediary, and direct-contract model plans that contract with individual physicians in the community.

Never event—A medical error that occurs in a facility (hospital or ambulatory surgical center) that should never happen. An example of a never event is amputation of the wrong limb. Definitions exist for 27 such never events. Medicare and most payers will not pay for care required as a result of a never event.

NIO—Non–investor owned. A term preferred by some not-for-profit health plans, including some Blue Cross and Blue Shield plans, because they are taxed as though they are for-profit health insurance companies, not as though they are charitable organizations.

Nonadmitted asset—An asset owned by an MCO that does not count toward its net worth by the insurance department. It varies from state to state but usually is applied to assets that cannot be readily converted into cash in the event of a health plan failure. It may also apply to only a portion of such an asset; for example, no more than 5% of a plan's net worth can consist of such assets as computers, real estate, and so forth.

Non-par—Short for nonparticipating. Refers to a provider that does not have a contract with the health plan.

NPI—National provider identifier. The NPI is mandated under HIPAA and replaced almost all other types of provider (broadly defined) identifiers regardless of customer (i.e., commercial health plan, Medicare, Medicaid, TRICARE, and so forth). The NPI is a 10-digit number and contains no embedded intelligence; that is, it contains no information about the health care provider such as the type of health care provider or state where the health care provider is located. The NPI does not replace the DEA number or the tax ID number of a provider, however.

NPlanID–The National Health Plan Identifier mandated under HIPAA. These will be the identifiers used by health plans (broadly defined) when conducting all transactions, regardless of the type of customer (e.g., commercial health plan, Medicare plan, and so forth) or provider. At the time of publication, neither the standards for the NPlanID nor an implementation date have been announced. The actual name for this identifier may change when it is finally defined.

OIG—The Office of the Inspector General. This is the federal agency responsible for conducting investigations and audits of federal contractors or any system that receives funds or reimbursement from the federal government. There are actually several OIG departments in different federal programs; examples pertinent to managed health care include TRICARE, CMS, and the FEHBP.

Open access—A term that refers to an HMO that does not use a primary care physician gatekeeper model for access to specialty physicians. In other words, a member may self-refer to a specialty physician rather than seeking an authorization from the PCP. HMOs that use an open-access model often have a significant copayment differential between care received. May also be called direct access.

Open enrollment period—The period when an employee may change health plans; this usually occurs once per year. A general rule is that most managed care plans will have around half their membership up for open enrollment in the fall for an effective date of January 1. A special form of open enrollment is still law in some states. This yearly open enrollment requires an HMO to accept any individual applicant (i.e., one not coming in through an employer group) for coverage regardless of health status. Such special open enrollments usually occur for 1 month each year. Many Blue Cross Blue Shield plans have similar open enrollments for indemnity products.

Open-panel HMO—A managed care plan that contracts (either directly or indirectly) with private physicians to deliver care in their own offices. Examples include a direct contract HMO and an IPA.

OPL—Other party liability. See COB.

Outlier—Something that is well outside of an expected range. May refer to a provider who is using medical resources at a much higher rate than his or her peers, to a case in a hospital that is far more expensive than anticipated, to a

Medicare inpatient who is far more costly than expected under the DRG, or in fact to anything at all that is significantly more or less than expected.

Outsourcing—Having a process or activity that an MCO provides done by a contracted third party. For example, contracting with an offshore company to manually enter data from images of paper claims.

OWA—Other weird arrangement. Refers to some type of benefits plan, product design, network contract, or whatever, that some bright person or consultant has cooked up but for which there is no precedent and no track record.

P4P—See Pay for performance.

Par provider—Shorthand term for participating provider (i.e., one who has signed an agreement with a plan to provide services). May apply to professional or institutional providers.

Part D—The drug benefit created under the MMA. May be provided by a private, freestanding prescription drug plan or included in an MA plan.

Pay for performance—The term applied to providing financial incentives to providers (hospitals and/or physicians) to improve compliance with standards of care and to improve outcomes and patient safety. Usually referred to as P4P in print.

PBM—See Pharmacy Benefit Manager.

PCCM—Primary care case manager. This acronym is used in Medicaid managed care programs and refers to the state designating PCPs as case managers to function as gatekeepers, but reimbursing those PCPs using traditional Medicaid fee for service and paying the PCP a nominal management fee, such as $2–$5 PMPM.

PCP—Primary care physician. Generally applies to internists, pediatricians, family physicians, and general practitioners, and occasionally to obstetrician/gynecologists.

PDP—Prescription drug plan. A private, freestanding plan providing drug coverage to Medicare beneficiaries under MA. Does not provide coverage for other services.

Pended/suspended claims—Although the terms "pend" and "suspend" are often used synonymously, some MCOs differentiate between claims that examiners place on hold (pends) and those that are placed on hold automatically by one or more systems edits (suspends).

PEPM—Per employee per month. Like PMPM, but roles up the unit to the level of the employee or subscriber rather than measuring based on all members (subscriber plus dependents).

Per diem reimbursement—Reimbursement of an institution, usually a hospital, based on a set rate per day rather than on charges. Per diem reimbursement can be varied by service (e.g., medical/surgical, obstetrics, mental health, and intensive care) or can be uniform regardless of intensity of services.

Persistency—Also called a persistency ratio. The term refers to a commercial group staying with an MCO from year to year. A persistency ratio of 90 would mean that 90% of groups enrolled do not change health plans.

Personal health record (PHR)—A record, usually created by a health plan, of an individual's health-related data. The sources of that data include claims from providers, prescription drugs that the plan paid for, demographic data, and so forth. Clinical data such as results of diagnostic lab or imaging, may be provided if the plan has access to it, and the member can add additional data, such as drug allergies or the results of a health risk appraisal. The purpose is to provide at least a usable subset of important health-related information in an electronically portable or transmittable format to improve continuity of care and emergency care.

PFFS—See Private fee-for-service plan.

Pharmacy Benefit Manager (PBM)—An independent company or subsidiary of an MCO that manages the pharmacy benefit, including pricing, paying the pharmacies, determining the levels of coverage of various drugs, and so forth.

PHI—Protected health information. Information that reveals medical information or data about an individual. PHI is addressed specifically by HIPAA in the Privacy and Security sections.

PHO—Physician-hospital organization. These are legal (or perhaps informal) organizations that bond hospitals and the attending medical staff and were developed for the purpose of contracting with managed care plans. A PHO may be open to any members of the staff who apply, or they may be closed to staff members who fail to qualify (or who are part of an already overrepresented specialty).

PHR—See Personal health record.

Physician incentive program—A generic term referring to a reimbursement methodology under which a physician's income from an MCO (or an IDS) is affected by the physician's performance or the overall performance of the plan (e.g., utilization, medical cost, quality measurements, member satisfaction, and so forth). This term has a very specific usage by the CMS, which limits the degree of incentive or risk allowed under a Medicare HMO (refer to PIP regulations at 42 CFR 422.208/210 of the June 26, 1998, regulations that implement Medicare Part C). CMS essentially bans "gainsharing" via a PIP altogether in an IDS receiving reimbursement under Medicare. Some states also now have laws and regulations regarding limits on PIPs and requirements for disclosure of incentives to members enrolled in MCOs. See also SFR.

PMPM—Per member per month. Specifically applies to a revenue or cost for each enrolled member (subscribers and dependents both) each month.

PMPY—Per member per year. The same as PMPM, but based on a year.

POS—Point of service. A plan in which members do not have to choose how to receive services until they need them. The most common use of the term applies to a plan that enrolls each member in both an HMO (or HMO-like) system and a PPO or an indemnity plan. These plans provide a difference in benefits (e.g., 100% coverage rather than 70%) depending on whether the member chooses to use the plan (including its providers and in compliance with the authorization system) or go outside the plan for services.

PPMC—Physician practice management company. An organization that manages a physician's practices, and in most cases either owns the practices outright or has rights to purchase them in the future. PPMCs concentrate only on physicians and not on hospitals, although some PPMCs have also branched into joint ventures with hospitals and insurers. Most PPMCs failed spectacularly, but some still exist, particularly for single specialties.

PPO—Preferred provider organization. A plan that contracts with independent providers at a discount for services. The panel is limited in size and usually has some type of utilization review system associated with it. A PPO may be risk bearing, like an insurance company, or may be non–risk bearing, like a physician-sponsored PPO that markets itself to insurance companies or self-insured companies via an access fee.

PPS—See Prospective payment system.

Preauthorization—See Authorization. See also Precertification.

Precertification—Also known as preadmission certification, preadmission review, and pre-cert. The process of obtaining certification or authorization from the health plan for routine hospital admissions or for ambulatory procedures. Often involves appropriateness review against criteria and assignment of length of stay. Failure to obtain precertification often results in a financial penalty to either the provider or the subscriber.

Preexisting condition—A medical condition for which a member has received treatment during a specified period of time prior to becoming covered under a health plan. May have an effect on whether treatments for that condition will be covered under certain types of health plans.

Premium—The money paid to a health plan for coverage. The term may be applied on an individual basis or a group basis.

Premium tax—A tax levied by a state on health insurance premiums for policies sold in that state. Employers that self-fund their health benefits plan, as well as Medicare Advantage plans, are not subject to premium taxes.

Prepaid or prepayment—Payment for services before they are incurred. Capitation is a form of prepayment because the provider is paid before the month that services will be provided. HMOs were once called prepaid health plans because premiums were paid in advance of the HMO providing the service. Can also be applied to the prepayment of any type of insurance premium, though health plans sometimes prefer to call it unearned premium revenue. Never applies to self-funding except when self-funded plans fund capitation to providers.

Preventive care—Healthcare that is aimed at preventing complications of existing diseases or preventing the occurrence of a disease. Often misspelled as "preventative," which until recently was not even considered a word; don't use it.

Private fee-for-service (PFFS) plan—A type of Medicare Advantage plan in which a private insurance company accepts risk for enrolled beneficiaries but pays providers on a FFS basis that does not have any risk component to the provider. PFFS plans are not network plans in the sense of being able to limit coverage to a network and must cover the cost of care from any provider willing to accept the individual as a patient, consistent with the rules of the plan regarding coverage.

Private inurnment—What happens when a not-for-profit business operates in such a way as to provide more than incidental financial gain to a private individual—for example, if a not-for-profit hospital pays too much money for a physician's practice or fails to charge fair market rates for services provided to a physician. Prohibited by the IRS.

PRO—Peer review organization. The old name for organizations charged with reviewing quality and cost for Medicare. Since replaced by QIOs.

Profiling—Measuring a provider's performance on selected measures and comparing that performance with similar providers. Usually applied to physicians. May be used for purposes of network selection or tiering, feedback reports, and/or P4P programs. Very complicated to perform properly.

Prospective payment system (PPS)—Medicare's terminology for determining fixed pricing for reimbursement of hospitals and facilities for care. The best-known examples of PPSs are DRGs, APCs, and now MS-DRGs. Prospective payment may be used by commercial plans because it applies to payment of facilities using the same methodologies.

Prospective review—Reviewing the need for medical care before the care is rendered. Also see Precertification.

Provider—The generic term used to refer to anyone providing medical services. In fact, it may even be used to refer to any*thing* that provides medical services, such as a hospital. Most often, however, it is used to refer to physicians. How physicians migrated from being called physicians to being called providers is not very clear cut and certainly not embraced by physicians, but it is a term in general use, including in this book.

Prudent layperson—See Reasonable layperson standard.

PSO—Provider-sponsored organization. An entity allowed under the BBA '97 Medicare+Choice. A PSO is a risk-bearing managed care organization that contracts directly with CMS for Medicare enrollees, but unlike an HMO, the PSO is made up of the providers themselves, and the providers bear substantial risk for expenses. The rules for financial solvency are somewhat different for a PSO as compared with an HMO, and if a PSO is not licensed by the state, provisions exist to seek licensure directly from the CMS. PSOs are the result of the belief by providers and legislators that there were fat profits to be had by "cutting out the middle man" in the form of removing the HMO from the equation. A few PSOs actually got started under a demonstration program, and a few more came into being after being authorized in the Balanced Budget Amendment of 1997. Most failed utterly and are defunct, though a few remain.

PTMPY—Per thousand members per year. A common way of reporting utilization. The most common example is hospital utilization, expressed as days per thousand members per year.

QA or QM—Quality assurance (older term) or quality management (newer term).

QIO—See Quality improvement organization.

QIP—Quality Improvement Program. The program put in place by CMS for Medicare Advantage plans of all types. The QIP uses data from HEDIS, HOS, and CAHPS, as well as financial and member disenrollment data. Accreditation by NCQA is also considered under the QIP.

Quality improvement organization (QIO)—An organization under contract to CMS to conduct quality reviews of providers, respond to beneficiary complaints about care, measure and report performance of providers, ensure that payment is made only for medically necessary services, and other functions. Applies to all types of plans and services, not just managed care.

Rate—The amount of money that a group or individual must pay to the health plan for coverage. Usually a monthly fee. Rating refers to the health plan developing those rates.

RBC—See Risk-based capital.

RBRVS—Resource-based relative value scale. This is a relative value scale developed for the CMS for use by Medicare. The RBRVS assigns relative values to each CPT code for services on the basis of the resources related to the procedure rather than simply on the basis of historical trends. The practical effect has been to lower reimbursement for procedural services (e.g., cardiac surgery) and to raise reimbursement for cognitive services (e.g., office visits).

Reasonable layperson standard—This means that the judgment of a reasonable nonclinician should be applied in determining if a service is warranted. This standard is almost always focused on the use of emergency or urgent care, when a layperson has good reason to believe that a medical problem must be addressed immediately, even if a trained provider may not feel that it was urgent.

Reinstatement—When an insurance or managed care policy is reinstated after payment for delinquent premiums during a defined grace period. See Grace period.

Reinsurance—Insurance purchased by a health plan to protect it against extremely high cost cases (also see Stop-loss).

Rental PPO—A PPO network owned and managed by a third party that rents access (and often services such as claims repricing) to an MCO or health insurance company. Not the same as a risk-bearing PPO that combines a network with the insurance function.

Reserves—The amount of money that a health plan puts aside to cover health care costs. This may apply to anticipated costs such as IBNRs, or it may apply to money that the plan does not expect to have to use to pay for current medical claims but keeps as a cushion against future adverse health care costs. Reserves can only be made up of admitted assets. Also called statutory reserves because the accounting is done per statutory accounting principles (SAP), not generally accepted accounting principles (GAAP), allowing the state insurance department greater leeway in deciding what counts toward net worth based on the liquidity of the assets. See also Admitted asset, Nonadmitted asset, and Risk-based capital.

Retail care clinic—A small clinic, usually associated with a retail store such as a pharmacy or grocery store, staffed by nonphysician providers. These clinics diagnose and treat a variety of low-acuity medical conditions at costs that are substantially lower than what a physician would charge.

Retention—A term with two meanings depending on context. Retention is used to describe that portion of a health insurance premium that is for administrative costs, not medical claims cost. Retention may also be used as a synonym for persistency; see Persistency.

Retrospective review—Reviewing health care costs after the care has been rendered. There are several forms of retrospective review. One form looks at individual claims for medical necessity, billing errors, or fraud. The other form looks at patterns of costs rather than individual cases.

Rider—An add-on to the core insurance or HMO policy, for example, coverage for dental or optometry services. Surprisingly, most regular drug benefits are provided via a rider and are not part of the main medical-surgical policy, whereas coverage for injectable drugs (including specialty pharmacy drugs) may be part of the main policy.

Risk adjustment—A methodology to account for the health status of patients when predicting or explaining costs of health care for defined populations or for evaluating retrospectively the performance of providers who care for them. Also known as severity adjustment and acuity adjustment. Case mix is related but applies only to inpatient care.

Risk-based capital (RBC)—A formula embodied in the Risk-Based Capital for Health Organizations Model Act, created under the auspices of the NAIC. RBC takes into account the fluctuating value of plan assets; the financial condition of plan affiliates; the risk that providers may not be able to provide contracted services; the risk that amounts due may not be recovered from reinsurance carriers; and general business risks (i.e., expenses may exceed income). The RBC formula gives credit for provider payment arrangements that reduce underwriting risk, including capitation and provider withholds, bonuses, contracted fee schedules, and aggregate cost arrangements. Although not required in all states, RBC is the agreed-upon standard for an insurance department to determine whether a health plan meets minimum financial solvency requirements.

Risk contract—Also known as a Medicare Risk Contract. An informal term that was once commonly used, but less so now. A contract between a health plan and the CMS under Medicare Advantage, under which the health plan provides services to Medicare beneficiaries and receives a monthly payment for enrolled Medicare members on an at-risk basis.

Risk corridor—The upper and lower limits of financial risk for a health plan or provider that is at risk for medical costs. Both limits must exist to be considered a risk corridor. A risk corridor of 20 percent, for example, would mean that the plan or provider can have financial losses or gains of no more than 10 percent of the baseline payment.

Risk management—Management activities aimed at lowering an organization's legal and financial exposures, especially to lawsuits.

Risk pool—This term can have two different meanings as applied to managed care, though both are related to medical care costs. In one case, it refers to a pool of funds that may be drawn against to cover medical costs, with any unused funds being paid to a provider or providers under capitation. The other meaning refers to the group of individuals (e.g., employees or Medicare enrollees) for which premiums are paid to an MCO or health insurance company, the money paid by or on behalf of healthier people then being used to cover the costs of sicker people (i.e., spreading out the risk by pooling the money).

RVU—Relative value unit. A number used as a multiplier to calculate the payment to a provider. The RVU is determined based on the procedure, then used by a plan to multiply against a value for each RVU to determine total payment to the provider. Not consistent or uniform, the RVU is often a combination of negotiation and national standards. See also RBRVS.

Safe harbor—The circumstances under which a hospital or other health care entity can provide something to a physician or other health entity and not violate the antikickback portion of the Stark regulations. See Stark regulations.

Schedule of benefits—The listing of what is and what is not covered by a health plan, and under what circumstances.

SCHIP—State Children's Health Insurance Program. A program created by the federal government to provide a "safety net" and preventive-care level of health coverage for children, funded through a combination of federal and state funds and administered by the states, through Medicaid in conformance with federal requirements.

SCP—Specialty care physician (i.e., a physician who is not a PCP). SCP is not used as an acronym nearly as often as PCP is.

Second opinion—An opinion obtained from another physician regarding the necessity for a treatment that has been recommended by another physician. May be required by some health plans for certain high-cost procedures. Once commonly used, now uncommon.

Section 1115 waiver—That section of federal law that provides for a state to opt out of the standard Medicaid fee-for-service program and adopt a managed care approach to financing and providing health care services to Medicaid-eligible recipients. Usually requires that some of the savings be applied to broaden coverage of who is eligible for Medicaid.

Section 125 Plan—See Flexible benefits plan.

Self-insured or self-funded plan—A health plan in which the risk for medical cost is assumed by the company rather than an insurance company or managed care plan. Under ERISA, self-funded plans are exempt from state laws and regulations such as premium taxes and mandatory benefits. Self-funded plans often contract with insurance companies or third-party administrators to administer the benefits (also see ASO).

Service area—The geographic area in which an HMO provides access to primary care. The service area is usually specifically designated by the regulators (state or federal), and the HMO is prohibited from marketing outside the service area. May be defined by county or by ZIP code. It is possible for an HMO to have more than one service area and for the service areas to either be contiguous (i.e., they actually border each other) or noncontiguous (i.e., there is a geographic gap between the service areas).

Service bureau—A weak form of integrated delivery system in which a hospital (or other organization) provides services to a physician's practice in return for a fair market price. May also try to negotiate with managed care plans, but generally not considered to be an effective negotiating mechanism.

Service plan—A health insurance plan that has direct contracts with providers but is not necessarily a managed care plan. The archetypal service plans are traditional (i.e., non–managed care) Blue Cross and Blue Shield plans, though a few non-Blue service plans do exist. The contract applies to direct billing of the plan by providers (rather than billing of the member), a provision for direct payment of the provider (rather than reimbursement of the member), a requirement that the provider accept the plan's determination of UCR and not balance bill the member in excess of that amount, and a range of other terms. May or may not address issues of utilization and quality.

SFR—Significant financial risk. A term used by the CMS that refers to the total amount of a physician's income at risk in a Medicare HMO. Such financial risk is considered "significant" when it exceeds a certain percentage of the total potential income that physician could receive under the reimbursement program. SFR is most commonly defined as any physician incentive payment program that allows for a variation of more than 25% between the minimum and the maximum amount of potential reimbursement.

Shock claim—Also referred to as a catastrophic claim. A shock claim is an extraordinarily expensive total cost of health care for an individual patient. Shock claims are taken into account by actuaries when they determine the trends for medical costs because shock claims have a certain amount of randomness to them; they are infrequent and costly, unlike routine care that is predictable.

Silent PPO—A term that is now rarely used because it is considered unethical or illegal. A silent PPO was a form of rental PPO (see Rental PPO) that the MCO or health insurance company did not clearly identify was being used when a member received services (by having the PPO's logo on the ID card somewhere, for example). This led to unanticipated reductions in payments because PPO reimbursement policies were applied after the fact.

Single specialty hospital—A hospital that provides services focusing on a single specialty, such as cardiac procedures or orthopedics. Physicians often have a small equity interest in them.

Slice business—A term referring to more than one MCO or health insurance company offering plans to the employees of one company.

SNP—See Special needs plan.

Special needs plan—A type of MA plan. This type of plan may exclusively enroll, or enroll a disproportionate percentage of, special needs Medicare beneficiaries. Individuals with special needs include beneficiaries entitled to both Medicare and Medicaid (dual eligibles), institutionalized beneficiaries, and individuals with severe or disabling chronic conditions.

Specialty network manager—A term used to describe a single specialist (or perhaps a specialist organization) who accepts capitation to manage a single specialty. Specialty services are supplied by many different specialty physicians, but the network manager has the responsibility for managing access and cost, and is at economic risk. A relatively uncommon model.

Specialty pharmacy—Injectable drugs that are almost always proteins created through recombinant DNA. These specialty drugs (unlike insulin, which would otherwise meet the criteria) focus on relatively uncommon but very costly conditions. They also frequently have only one single source.

Specialty pharmacy distributor (SPD)—A company that distributes specialty pharmacy, from the manufacturer to the provider and/or directly to the patient, to address the unique distribution, storage, and utilization issues around these types of injectable drugs. May be part of a PBM or a separate company.

Staff model HMO—An HMO that employs providers directly, and those providers see members in the HMO's own facilities. A form of closed-panel HMO. A different use of this term is sometimes applied to vertically integrated health care delivery systems that employ physicians, but in which the system is not licensed as an HMO.

Stark regulations—Named after Fortney "Pete" Stark, congressional representative from California. The so-called Stark regulations are actually two sets of regulations: Stark I and Stark II, stemming from the Ethics in Referrals Act. These regulations are not for amateurs to handle, and competent legal counsel is required for any provider system doing business with federal or state governments.

State licensure—The license or certificate of authority issued by a state to a health plan that allows the plan to write business in the state. May be based on having a license in a different state; see State of domicile.

State of domicile—The state in which an insurance company or MCO is licensed as its primary location. For example, an MCO may have its state of domicile in Virginia but also be licensed and doing business in Maryland and the District of Columbia. In many states, the insurance commissioner will defer primary regulation to the insurance department in the state of domicile as long as all minimum standards of the state are met.

Statutory reserves—See Reserves.

Stop-loss—A form of reinsurance that provides protection for medical expenses above a certain limit, generally on a year-by-year basis. This may apply to an entire health plan or to any single component. For example, the health plan may have stop-loss reinsurance for cases that exceed $100,000. After a case hits $100,000, the plan receives 80 percent of expenses in excess of $100,000 back from the reinsurance company for the rest of the year. Another example would be the plan providing a stop-loss to participating physicians for referral expenses over $2,500. When a case exceeds that amount in a single year, the plan no longer deducts those costs from the physician's referral pool for the remainder of the year. Specific coverage refers to individual cases, whereas aggregate coverage refers to the total costs rather than a specific case.

Subacute care facility—A health facility that is a step down from an acute care hospital. May be a nursing home or a facility that provides medical care but not surgical or emergency care. Some confine use of the term to services that are a step up from the conventional skilled nursing facility intensity of services, adding RNs around the clock and intravenous medications.

Subrogation—The contractual right of a health plan to recover payments made to a member for health care costs after that member has received such payment for damages in a legal action.

Subscriber—The individual or member who has the health plan coverage by virtue of being eligible on his or her own behalf rather than as a dependent.

Sutton's law—"Go where the money is!" Attributed to the Depression-era bank robber Willie Sutton, who, when asked why he robbed banks, replied, "That's where the money is." Sutton apparently denied ever having made that statement. In any event, it is a good law to use when determining what needs attention in a managed care plan.

Taft-Hartley plan—A type of health plan provided by a union to its members, usually using funds contributed by more than one employer or company. Also eligible to be a type of MA plan.

TANF—Temporary Assistance to Needy Families. Administered by DHHS, TANF provides assistance and work opportunities to needy families by granting states the federal funds and wide flexibility to develop and implement their own welfare programs.

TAT—Turnaround time. The amount of time it takes a health plan to process and pay a claim from the time it arrives.

Termination date—The day that health plan coverage is no longer in effect.

Tiering—A term that applies to categorizing something into different tiers for purposes of benefits differentials. When used in pharmacy, Tier 1 drugs require lower copays than do Tier 2, Tier 3, and so forth. When applied to providers, members accessing Tier 1 providers likewise have less (or even no) cost sharing than if they use a Tier 2 provider.

Total capitation—See Global capitation.

TPA—Third-party administrator. A firm that performs administrative functions (e.g., claims processing, membership, and the like) for a self-funded plan or a start-up managed care plan (also see ASO).

Transparency—Refers to making data available to the public. Also called pricing transparency when such data involve the price for services from different providers of care.

Triage—The origins of this term are grisly: The process of sorting out wounded soldiers into those who need treatment immediately, those who can wait, and those who are too severely injured to even try and save (and therefore only made as comfortable as possible). In health plans, this refers to the process of sorting out requests for services by members into those who need to be seen right away, those who can wait a little while, and those whose problems can be handled with advice over the phone. Its use has diminished.

TRICARE—The Department of Defense's worldwide managed health care program. TRICARE was initiated in 1995, integrating health care services provided in the direct care system of military hospitals and clinics with services purchased from civilian providers for anybody eligible for coverage (e.g., retirees and dependents). There are various different TRICARE benefits programs. The portion of care provided under TRICARE by non-military hospitals and providers is administered by private managed care companies in three regions in the United States.

Triple option—The offering of an HMO, a PPO, and a traditional insurance plan by one carrier.

UB-92—See CMS-1450.

UCR—Usual, customary, or reasonable. A method of profiling prevailing fees in an area and reimbursing providers on the basis of that profile. One archaic method is to average all fees and choose the 80th or 90th percentile, although in this era, a plan will usually use another method to determine what is reasonable. Sometimes this term is used synonymously with a fee allowance schedule when that schedule is set relatively high.

Unbundling—The practice of a provider billing for multiple components of service that were previously included in a single fee. For example, if dressings and instruments were included in a fee for a minor procedure, the fee for the procedure remains the same, but there are now additional charges for the dressings and instruments.

Underwriting—In one definition, this refers to bearing the risk for something (i.e., a policy is underwritten by an insurance company). In another definition, this refers to the analysis of a group to determine rates and benefits or to determine whether the group should be offered coverage at all. A related definition refers to health screening of each individual applicant for insurance and refusing to provide coverage for preexisting conditions.

Upcoding—The practice of a provider billing for a procedure that pays better than the service actually performed. For example, an office visit that would normally be reimbursed at $45 is coded as one that is reimbursed at $53.

UPIN—Universal provider identification number. An identification number once issued by CMS for use in billing Medicare. The UPIN was replaced by the NPI in 2007 and is no longer in use. See NPI.

URAC—A not-for-profit organization that performs reviews on external utilization review agencies (freestanding companies, utilization management departments of insurance companies, or utilization management departments of managed care plans). Its primary focus is MCOs, though they have expanded their accreditation activities—for example, accrediting health-related Web sites. States often require certification by URAC or another accreditation organization to operate. URAC once stood for the Utilization Review Accreditation Commission but now is only known as URAC.

URO—Utilization review organization. A freestanding organization that does nothing but UR, usually on a remote basis, using the telephone and paper correspondence. It may be independent or part of another company, such as an insurance company that sells UR services on a stand-alone basis.

Worker's compensation—A form of social insurance provided through property-casualty insurers. Worker's compensation provides medical benefits and replacement of lost wages that result from injuries or illnesses that arise from the workplace; in turn, the employee cannot normally sue the employer unless true negligence exists. Worker's compensation has undergone dramatic increases in cost as group health has shifted into managed care, resulting in worker's compensation carriers adopting managed care approaches. Worker's compensation is often heavily regulated under state laws that are significantly different from those used for group health insurance, and it is often the subject of intense negotiation between management and organized labor.

Index

Italics indicate appearance within a table or figure; 'n' indicates appearance within a footnote.

A

C

Designated Standards Maintenance Organizations (DSMOs), 188, 217
diabetes, *202*
"diagnosis-procedure" mismatch, 137
diagnosis-related groups (DRGs), 78–79, 219
diagnostic ancillary services, 86–89, 106–107
Diagnostic and Statistical Manual of Mental Disorders, 4th edition (DSM-IV), 219
differential by day in hospital, 78
direct contract models, 33, 217
direct contracting, 217–218
direct corporate liability, 183
direct-pay subscribers, 218
direct-to-consumer advertising, 90
directors of information services, 49–50
disabled persons, Medicare coverage, 156
discharge facilitation, 101, 218
discounted charges
    ancillary services, 88, 107–108
    behavioral health services, 111–112
    features of, 77
    for insurers, 30
    outpatient procedures, 83
    prescriptions, 109, 110
disease management (DM), 10, 36–37, 104–106, 218
disenrollment, *130*, 218
disincentives, 97
dispense as written (DAW), 216
dispensing fees, 218
disputes, 140. *See also* coverage denial
distribution, 121–123, *122*
distribution channels, 218
District of Columbia, 103
District of Columbia Medical Society, 3
divorce, 185
DM (disease management), 10, 36–37, 104–106, 218
DME (durable medical equipment), 218
DNA replication, 15
DO (doctor of osteopathy), 60
doctor of chiropractic (DC), 60
doctor of osteopathy (DO), 60
DOH (department of health), 176

DOI (department of insurance), 176, 178
DOL (U.S. Department of Labor), 25, 35, 181, 195, 219
Donabedian, Avedis, 113
doughnut holes, 35, 158, 219
DRGs (diagnosis-related groups), 78–79, 219
Drug Enforcement Administration (DEA), 66, 68, 191
drug store clinics, 61
drug utilization reviews (DURs), 89–90, 109–110, 111, 219
drugs. *See* prescriptions
drugstore chains, 90
DSM-IV (*Diagnostic and Statistical Manual of Mental Disorders*, 4th edition), 219
DSMOs (Designated Standards Maintenance Organizations), 188, 217
dual-choice provisions, 5, 6
dual eligibles, 157, 158, 167, 174, 219
"due process" termination requirements, 51, 59
"dumping" (of uninsured patients), 82
duplication, claims, 139
durable medical equipment (DME), 218
DURs (drug utilization reviews), 89–90, 109–110, 111, 219

E

EAPs (employee assistance programs), 112, 219
economy, healthcare impact, 11–12, 15
ED (emergency department). *See* emergency department (ED)
EDI (electronic data interchange), 219
effective date, 220
efficiency, 140
EFT (electronic funds transfer), 139, 220
EINs (National Employer Identification Numbers), 191
electronic connectivity. *See also* Internet
    online sales, 123
    physician network management, 68

urgent care claims. *See* "expedited reviews"
UROs (utilization review organizations), 250
U.S. Department of Health and Human
    Services (HHS). *See* Health and
    Human Services (HHS)
U.S. Department of Health, Education and
    Welfare. *See* Health and Human
    Services (HHS)
U.S. Department of Labor (DOL), 25, 35,
    181, 195, 219
U.S. Public Health Service, 19
U.S. Supreme Court, 3, 179
U.S. Treasury Department, 35
use. *See* utilization management (UM)
use of services, 201, *203*
usual, customary, or reasonable (UCR), 29,
    72, 249
Utah, 171
utilization management (UM). *See also*
    benefits design
  components of, *98*, 98–102
  contractual requirements, 57
  features of, 26
  fee incentives, 72
  HEDIS measures, 201, *203*
  incentive payments, 70
  indemnity insurance, 29
  services, 201
Utilization Review Accreditation
    Commission. *See* URAC
Utilization Review Model Act, 178
utilization review organizations (UROs), 250
utilization reviews
  committees, 52
  history of, 6

HMO, 32
indemnity insurance, 26, 29
  of inpatient care, 10
  of physician incentives, 70, 72, 165

V
vaginal deliveries, 186
Veterans Administration, 19
vicarious liability, 183
"viral cocktail" regimens, 90
volume (utilization)
  discounts, 77, 78, 88
  prescriptions, 109, 110
  pricing vs., 95

W
waiting periods for coverage, 195
waivers, cost sharing, 97
Washington State, 1, 3, 4
Web sites, xvii, 163, 165
welfare reform legislation, 170
wellness programs, 97
WellPoint, 12
Western Clinic, 1
whole dollars, 145
wholesale versus retail, *124*, 124–125
withholds, 70, 72, 73–74, 100
Women's Health and Cancer Rights Act of
    1998, 186
work site wellness programs, 7
worker's compensation, 250
working spouses, 127, 138
wraparound policies, 21, 23–24